॥ओ३म्॥

Āyurved

Its Principles & Philosophies

Acharya Balkrishna

॥ओ३म्॥

Publisher : **DIVYA PRAKASHAN**
Divya Yog Mandir Trust
Patanjali Yogpeeth,
Delhi-Hardwar Road, Bahadarabad
Hardwar – 249 408 (Uttarakhand)

E mail : divyayoga@rediffmail.com
Website : www.divyayoga.com
Telephone : 91-1334-244107, 240008, 246737
Fax : 91-1334-244805

Second Edition : 10,000 Copies (July 2007)

Printer : **Sai Security Printers Pvt. Limited**
152, DLF Industrial Area Faridabad -121003 (Haryana)
Phone : 0129-2276370, 2272277, Fax : 0129-2256239
E mail : sspdel@saiprinters.com

Distributor : **Diamond Pocket Books (Pvt.) Ltd.**
X-30, Okhla Industrial Area, Phase-II, New delhi-110020
Phone : 011-41611861, Fax : 011-41611866
Email : sales@diamondpublication.com
Website : www.diamondpublication.com

Price :

ISBN : 81-89235-56-7

301 (02-08)

FOREWORD

Amongst all the cultures of the world, Indian culture is not only ancient but also unique. *Vedas* are the root and basis of our culture and civilization, and are some of the oldest scriptures in the library of human beings. There are four *Vedas* : *Rigveda, Yajurveda, Saamveda* and *Atharved*. *Ayurved* is the oldest treatise related to treatment and health, it is believed to be a part of *Atharved* : This book is being presented to give useful and reliable information about the mysteries of the principles of the oldest and greatest treatise on ayurved.

The ancient learned sages described *Ayurved* as immortal. In support of their statement they have given three reasons which cannot be ruled out, these are –

"Soyaamaayurvedah shaashvato nirdishyate, anaaditvaat, Swbhaavsamsidhlakshantwaat, bhaavswbhaav nityatvaachh"

(Charak Samhita-Percept 30/26)

That which is Ayurved is in itself complete, eternal and immortal within itself. It regulates the behaviour of the mind and emotions. It is this immortal treatise on *Ayurved*, which was studied by *Prajapati* through *Brahma*, studied by princes of *Ashwani* through *Prajapati*, from whom *Indra* studied and from *Indra* the sage *Bhardwaj* studied it and passed on its knowledge to other sages like *Punarvasu, Aatreya, Agnivesh, Jatukarna, Parashar, Haareet, Shar Paani, Sushrut, Dhanvantri, Vaagbhat* and other worth quoting names .

In Indian culture, the four main valorous objectives of human life are to follow *dharm, arth, kaam, moksh* - duty, wealth, desire and salvation, and attain self-realization to get freedom from the cycle of birth and death and become closer to God. The actual basis of the attainment and accomplishment of the four kinds of valour is a healthy body because **"*Shareermaadhyam khalu dharma saadhanam*"**, according to which, the means that one can abide to one's duty only in a healthy body. If a person is healthy and free from disease then that person can follow the daily routine properly, perform his daily work and he even work hard. He can derive pleasure from any means of joy, earn his living by any enterprise or business, and serve the family, society and the nation, to practice and worship God for welfare of the self. It is because of this, that having a healthy body is the first of the seven pleasures that have been stated. *Ayurved* also states the same –

"Dharmarth kaamamokshanaam aarogyam moolmuttamam"

(Charak Samhita-Percept 1/15)

which means that health is the basis of duty, wealth, desire and salvation.

The importance and utility of the treatise on *Ayurved* has been questioned – **"*Kimarthmaayurvedah*"** which means- what is the objective of *Ayurved*? The answer is -

"Prayojanam chaasya swasthasya swaasthyarakshanmaaturasya vikaarprashmanamam cha"

(Charak Samhita-Percept 30/26)

The objective of *Ayurved* is to protect the health of a person and cure the diseases of a sick person. The most important thing is that this objective of *Ayurved* has not been created for earning profit or fame but is for the benefit of humanity with the feeling of kindness and compassion, that is-

"Dharmaartham chaarth kaamaarthmaayurvedo maharishibhih prakaashito dharma paraerichhdabhiah sthanamakshram"

(*Charak Samhita-Treatment* 1-4/57*)

This means that the sages engaged in religious activities and desirous of attaining salvation propagated the knowledge of *Ayurved* as their duty towards the religion, and not for fulfillment of any specific desire.The practitioner of *Ayurved* has been defined as-

"Naathaartha naapi kaamaatharthamatha bhoot dyaam prati vartate yashchikitsaayaam sa sarvmativartate"

(*Charak Samhita Chikitsaa* 1-4/58*)

The best doctor is the *vaidya* who performs his duty without seeking any specific desire, and only out of sympathy for the person (patient).

Ayurved is a practices of the principles of high idealism. It is an exceptional system of medicine which lays significant emphasis on the diet, that is, what to eat and what not to eat and describes that the means of eradication of the cause of the disease is the first step to cure that disease.

"Sanksheptaha kriyaa yogo nidaan parivarjanam" which means that first of all eliminate the cause of the disease. To prove its objectives *Ayurved* describes the ways and means to safeguard the health and also the reasons because of which diseases develop in the body.

Explaining the means of safeguarding health, *Ayurved* says -

"Traya upastambha iti – aahaaramah swapno brahmacharyamiti"

(*Charak Samhita-Percept 11/35*)

It means that *ahaar, swapna, bramacharya* i.e. food, sleep and celibacy are the three pillars that support stability, firmness and perfection of the body. By utilization of these three assisting pillars in accordance with the prescribed method, body and health can be safeguarded.

Alongwith this the causes of sickness have been discussed, that is-

"Ghee dhriti smriti veebhrashtah karmayat kurute ashubham pragyaparaadham tam vidyat sarvadosh prakopnam"

(*Charak Samhita-Shareer 1/102*)

It means that when a person performs inauspicious activities that destroy *Dhee* (brain), *dhriti* (patience) and *smriti* (memorizing power), then all the physical and mental defects become irate. These inauspicious deeds are called intellectual offences. One who commits intellectual offences, his body and health will suffer and he will be disease struck.

Ayurved while describing itself says-

"Tadayurveda yateetyaayurvedah"

(*Charak Samhita-Percept 30/23*)

which means that one who imparts knowledge about duration of life is known as *Ayurved*. It is also said-

"Hitaahitam sukham dukhmaayustasya hitaahitammaanam cha tachh yatroktamaayurvedah sa uchayate"

(Charak Samhita-Percept 1/41)

which means that the scripture in which diet to be taken and diet not to be taken, to honour or dishonour a duration and the appearance of the duration for the four kinds of durations i.e. good duration of life, bad duration of life, happy duration of life and unhappy duration of life has been described, is called *Ayurved*. Actually, *Ayurved* is the name given to an optimal and healthy life-style. It is the name of the knowledge of life and the science which makes human life healthy and happy. We can conclude that *Ayurved* is not merely the science that gives knowledge of treatments through herbal medicines and shrubs but an instruction & view of living a complete human life.

Medicines have been described not only for the well being of the ill but also for helping a healthy person to maintain and safeguard his health. The daily and the seasonal routines described give detailed information about the food-habits which are appropriate and beneficial as per the three constitutions of *vaat*, *pitta* and *kapha*. Descriptions have been given about the eatables that are mutually incompatable and unsuitable for consumption. Also mentioned are the micro- forces borne in the body. Actually it is a fact that *Ayurved* is such a vast subject that it can not be bound within a boundary. In *Ayurved* green plants, leaves, seeds, fruits etc. are considered as medicines. That is-

"Anenopdeshen naanaushadhi bootam jagati kimchid dravyamupalabhyate taam taam yuktimarth ch tam tambhipretya"

(Charak Samhita-Percept 26/12)

This means that, in this universe there is no such liquid which is not a medicine. According to different uses as per the requirement every substance functions as a medicine and each mineral can be purified and used as medicine, that can be life saving. Along with this, *Ayurved* also gives us knowledge about that intake of diet, lifestyle, consuming water and air in a systematic way increases longevity, knowledge about nature, soul and God. It gives guidance in overcoming the cycle of life and death to attain salvation. This knowledge presented by our learned sages proves beneficial for the lives of human beings and there is no doubt today that it needs to be spread to every nook and corner of this universe. New experiments and research in this field are required so that the treatment by this system can be done confidently. Even today there are capable *Ayurvedic* doctors, who are working with traditional methods. They are experienced and are able to cure diseases which are thought to be incurable, but due to lack of interaction, communication and assistance between them, utilization of *Ayurved* is not taking place universally.

We have established Brahmkalp *Chikitsalya* to serve millions of patients with the knowledge of *Ayurved* and have already cured many. We believe that research in *Ayurved* with modern technological updates is mandatory. This necessity has been understood in depth by Swami Ramdevji, under whose leadership, the preachings of *Ayurved* on the subjects of health, appropriate lifestyle, dietary habits, actions and thoughts etc., are being publicised and propagated by the Divya Yog Mandir Trust & Patanjali Yogpeeth.

Today human beings are distanced from nature and from their own intellect.This deprives them of the natural state of health. Guidance from *Ayurved* is necessary to retrieve the healthy body, pure mind and intellect because it is *Ayurved* which links the human beings with nature and with his own intellect within to give rise to inner knowledge about the best lifestyle. This book is being presented to make everyone aware of the strange, deep seated and unprecedented mysteries of *Ayurved*.

Sister Kanchan, the disciple of Vaidya Bhagwan Das has given us assistance in writing this book. After studying the *Ayurvedic* scriptures in depth she has collected their gist. I express my heartfelt thanks to her.

After processing this text on computer, it was sent to Dr. Premdutt Pandey, the chief editor of '*Nirogadham*', at Indore for proof reading and necessary corrections. Despite his busy schedule he submitted the book in time. This is evidence of his heartfelt affection and active assistance. I thank Dr.Pandey for his assistance.

I also thank and bless all the assistants, junior and senior doctors of the *ashram* who gave their assistance in writing of this book. May God give them sincere desire and interest in serving others ! In the end, I bow to my elder brother, the revered Swami Ramdevji Maharaj, who has been the source of inspiration for me in carrying out the services at the *ashram.* He has been providing me active assistance and it is due to his blessings that I am able to perform my duties. All my success and achievements are the result of his efforts. Swamiji is the representative of those learned sages of *Ayurved*, by whose efforts the knowledge of *Ayurved* is being propagated all over. I am grateful and bow down to all the learned sages who have protected, added and expanded the *Ayurvedic* scriptures. We should take the oath to propagating, securing and following the path of spirituality, *Ayurved, Yog* and *Vedic* tradition. We must have a firm faith that we will be blessed and be assisted by everyone in this sacred task.

Acharya Balkrishna

MY FEELINGS TOWARDS THE BOOK

When Acharya Balkrishna called me over phone and told me that he has authored a book entitled "*Ayurved- Its Principles & Philosophies*", and he is sending the same to me. He wanted that I may carry out any amendments or corrections that may be required in the book. Alongwith this he wanted me to carry out the proof reading of the matter and carryout corrections if any. Inspite of my busy schedule, I happily accepted the offer. By way of the magazine '*Nirogadham*' I have been interested and related to the activities and programmes of Swami Ramdevji Maharaj and have been assisting him as per my capabilities. It is due to this feeling, in no time, I accepted the offer to serve the teacher and preacher, and immediately accepted the proposal from Acharya Shri Balkrishan, who is the main coordinator and incharge of the activities and programmes being run by Swami Ramdevji.

When I received the book for proof reading, I was surprised to see that great effort has been put in collection and writing the contents of book. To prove each and every fact mentioned in the book, verses from the related *Ayurvedic* scriptures which have been quoted. Footnotes mentioning name of the scriptures, which have been given at the end of the page, so that the reader of the book may not experience any difficulty in referring to the verses mentioned therein.

The speciality of this book is that it includes in abundance all those things which are required in the life of a person. As this book is based on *Ayurved* therefore a number of instances and principles have been incorporated into it efficiently. The second speciallty about this book is that the language used in the book is very simple and interesting therefore a layman can also understand the contents of the book. The book is described in detail which give a clear view to the meanings. Sanskrit *shlokas* are inserted which increase the utility and importance of this book. I believe that the book is full of principles and rules of *Ayurved* and will soon be a part of every home in our country and the people of our country will read it and get benefited from it. I extend my heartiest good wishes that this book gets good appreciation in India and abroad and many editions of this book are published for the benefit of the society.

Wishing you good luck.

RAS Vaidya Dr. Premdutt Pandey
Chief Editor – *Nirogadham*

Contents

Contents

Introduction

1. What is *Āyuṛved*[1]?

All of us in general at some time or the other, have observed and realized that not only human beings but even the tiniest forms of life strive to survive, escape from sorrow and remain happy[2]. Ever since man was created, he has been engaged in a continuous struggle to fulfil his natural needs like hunger, thirst, sleep etc. and ward off diseases. *Āyuṛved* has its genesis in this context. Today, Allopathy, Homeopathy, Naturopathy, Reiki and many other systems of treatment claim to cure ailments. However, *Āyuṛved* is closest to our hearts. People suffering from stomach upset or acidity are advised to use *ajwāin* (thyme) and *hēeṇg* (asafoetida) and avoid drinking cold water and use remedies like ginger (*aḍrak*), holy basil (*tulsi*), tea, black pepper, and honey mixed in gingerjuice and turmeric powder with milk when they suffer from common cold, throat infection or cough[3]. Each spice or food material is 'hot' or 'cold', such *Āyuṛvedic* concepts have percolated through generations. Most of the ingredients of these home remedies are available in Indian kitchens and gardens and can be used as medicines. Thus *Āyuṛved* is an integral part

---

1. *Saṭvamāṭmā Śarēeraṃ ḉha trayametaṭtridanḍavaṭ*
Lōkaṣtiṣṭhaṭi Sanyogāttara sarvaṃ pratiṣṭhitaṃ
Sa Pamanṣ̌ḉetanaṃ taççha taççhaḍhikarnaṃ ṣmritaṃ
Vadaṣyāṣya ṭadarthaṃ Saṃprakāśitah (*Charak. Su. 1/46-47*)

2. *Ṗrayojanaṃ ḉhāsya ṣwaṣthaṣya ṣwāṣṭhyarakṣanaṃ*
āaturaṣya vikārpraśmaṇaṃ ḉha (*Charak. su. 30/26*)
Eha khalyāyuṛvēda ṗrayojanaṃ-Vyāḍhyupṣṛiṣṭānāṃ
Vyāḍhiparimokṣah ṣwaṣṭhaṣya rakṣaṇaṃ ḉha (*Su. Su. 1/22*)

3. *Sahṣravedhi jatukaṃ bāhikaṃ hiṅgu rāmathaṃ*
Hiṇguṣ̌ṇāṃ pāçanaṃ rūçyaṃ tēekṣanaṃ vātabalāsanuṭ
Śūlagulṃodarānāhakrimighnaṃ piṭtavarḍhanaṃ
Ṣtrīpuṣpajananaṃ balyaṃ mōorççhāpaṣmarahṛiṭ paraṃ (*Bha. pra.*)
Roḉhanaṃ dēepanaṃ ṿriśyaṃ āṛḍrakaṃ viṣ̌vaḅheṣajaṃ
Vātāṣ̌leṣmavibanḍhēśu rasaṣtaṣyōpadiśyatē (*Ch. su. 27/166*)
Nāgaraṃ kaphavātāghnaṃ vipākaṃ madhuraṃ kaṭu
Ṿriśyōṣnaṃ rochanaṃ saṣnēhaṃ laghudēepanaṃ (*Su. Su. 46/226*)
Yavānī kaṭutēekṣ̌ṇōṣ̌ṇā vātaṣ̌leṣmaḍvijāmayāṇ
hanti gulṃodaraṃ śōolaṃ dēepayāṭyaśu ḉhānalaṃ (*Dh Nig*)
Tulṣi laghuṛuṣṇā ḉh rōokṣā kaphvināśinī
ḳrimidośaṃ nishaṇtyeśā ruḉhikṛiṭ bahṿidēepanī (*Dh. Nig.*)

of our life.

It is logical to ascertain and try to comprehend what *Āyuṛved* really is. Etymologically the word *Āyuṛved* is combination of two words: *Ayush* which means life and *veda* which means knowledge, Hence *Āyuṛved* means 'Knowledge of Life[4]'. Simply stated, it embodies the art of living and is not only confined to knowledge about illnesses and their remedies. It provides comprehensive knowledge to enable one to lead a simple, productive and healthy life. The popular notion that *Āyuṛved* is only a system of medicine, because it gives systematic and organized information about health and illnesses, is severely limiting and incomplete.

Āyuṛved is the science that imparts not just the physical, but also the psychological and spiritual well-being of all living beings[5]. Defining *Āyuṛved*, in *Çharak Saṃhitā*, *Mahaṛishi Çharak* said, "The science that teaches us what is good or bad, what causes joy or sorrow, the duration and characteristics of life, is *Āyurved*[6]." It is evident, that *Āyuṛveda* is beneficial not only to a specific group of individuals, religion or country, but has immense universal significance. Just as life is real, so are *āyurvedic* principles and philosophies. They are valid wherever there is life. They are eternal and ever lasting[7]. The aim of these principles is to guide us to universal well-being and joy.

2. Unique features of *Āyuṛvedic* treatment

While treating with the *āyuṛvedic* system of medicine certain basics are borne in mind. This system of healing has certain peculiarities. A brief description is as follows:

♦ A comprehensive cure

During treatment, the physician does not isolate his attention to just the affected parts of the body or the symptoms of the illness, in addition, he examines the patient's constitution, emotional state, spiritual and other conditions. He also takes into consideration the condition of excretions and blood etc[8]. This explains why patients suffering from the same disease are prescribed different remedies.

---

4. *Āyuśo vedaḥ Āyurvedaḥ Āyuraṣminṿidẏatēsnēnā vādẏyurvinḍateeṭyāyuṛvedaḥ* (Su. su. 1/23)
Āyuḥ śarēerenḍriya saṭvāṭma sanẏōgaḥ tadaṣmināyurvēdē viḍyatē jgyayatē anēnēti āyurvedah (Dalhaṇ)
5. *Āhuḥ śarēerenḍriyasāṭvāṭma sanẏogo ḍhāri jēevitaṃ* (Ch. su. 1/42)
6. *Hitāhitaṃ Sukhaṃ dukhamayuṣtasya hitāhitam Māanaṃ ça taççha yaṭrōktamāyuṛvedaḥ sa uçhayatē* (Ch. su. 1/41)
7. *Sōbyamāyuṛvedaḥ śaṣvato niṛdiśyatē Anādiṭwāṭ, ṣwabhāvasanṣidhlakṣaṇaṭwāṭ, ḅhāṣwaḅhāvaniṭyaṭvāççha* (Ch. su. 30/26)
8. *Dośadhātumalamūlaṃ hi śarēeraṃ* (Su. su. 15/3)

♦ Psycho-somatic nature of illnesses

According to *Āyuṛved*, no disease is only physiological or only psychological. Physical ailments affect the psyche and mental disturbances affect physical health . Therefore, the body and psyche cannot be separated and considered individually for treatment. This is the rationale behind treating every disease as a psycho-somatic disorder[9]. According to *Acharya Charak*, all diseases – whether *vātaj*, *piṭtaraj*, *kaphaj* or psychological- have one basic cause - mistakes committed with knowledge *(Pragyaparadh)*.

The use of *āyuṛvedic* remedies has gained validity and efficacy over several millenia from the experience of the *Riśhis*. Nature is the primary source of all *āyuṛvedic* medicines. All ingredients are from either plant origin (herbs, extracts, juices etc.) or from animal world (milk *ghēe* etc.). Metals that used also occur naturally. No chemicals are used in the preparation of these medicines and therefore there are no toxic side-effects.

The reason why Allopathic physicians have reservations regarding *ayuṛvedic* medicines is the ingredients. The concern is misplaced because even metạls and like copper (varn) and other toxic/poisonous vegetable products e.g. *kuchlā*, *bhilāwā*, *āak* etc are never used in their original form but are subjected to numerous natural processes, purified and made compatible with the chemicals in the body before use. Consequently, far from being harmful, they prove beneficial to the patient[10].

♦ Every medicine is a tonic

All *āyuṛvedic* medicines act as tonics by virtue of providing nutrition to the body and triggering restorative processes in the brain, which in turn leads to healing of the psyche and correcting the mental, psychological and

---

9. *Saṛvēbpi tu khalṿētēb bhip̣raṿriḍhāṣ c̣haṭwāro rogāḥ,*
paraṣparamanubaṇdhaṇti, na c̣hāṇyoṇyēṇ saḥa
saṇdēhamāpaḍyatē (Ch. su. 20/6)

Ēṛśyāśōkabhaya ḳrōdhamānḍveṣadayaśc̣ha ye
manovikārāṣtēbp̣yuḳtāḥ saṛvep̣ragyāparādhajāḥ (Ch.su. 7/52)

10. *Halāhalaḥ kālakuṭaḥ ṣriṇgkaśc̣ha p̣radēepanaḥ*
Sāurāṣ̈ṭriko ḅrahṃaputrō hāriḍraḥ saḳtūkaṣtathā (R. ta. 24/7-8)

Vaṭsanābha itijgyeyā viṣbhedāḥ nava
Laṇgatī viśamuṣṭiṣc̣ha karvēero jayā tathā (R.R.S. 10/84)

Nēelakaḥ kanakobṛkaṣc̣ha vaṛgo ḥyupaviśāṭmakāḥ
Ye duṛguṇā viśebśuḍhha tē ṣyuṛhēenā viśōḍhitē (Āa. p̣r. 6/47-48)

Taṣmaḍviśaṃ p̣rogēśu śoḍhitaṃ yojyeḍḍhiśaḳ
Rasakaṛmaṇī śaṣtobyaṃ taḍhabaṇḍhan avidhāvapi (R.R.S. 10/83)

Ayuḳṭyā sevitaśc̣hāyaṃ mārayaṭyēva niśc̣hitaṃ
Rase Rasāyanādāu c̣ha vaṭsanābhaḥ p̣raśaṣyatē (R.ta. 24/7-8)

Viśatiṇdukabēejaṃ tu p̣rayahaṃ pariśēetalaṃ
Nihaṇti kuḳkuraviśaṃ khalu māasāikamātrataḥ (R. ta. 24/30)

emotional imbalances. This unique restorative characteristic of *āyuṛvedic* medicines makes them useful even for people who are in good health. Thus, they are not only curative, but also nutritive and prophylactic as they strengthen the immune system. For exa mple- "*Chyawanprash*"[11], "*Chanḍra prabhavati*"[12] etc are some of the most common restorative-nutritive *āyuṛvedic* tonics.

♦ Importance of developing immune system and dietary control

In the *Āyuṛvedic* system of medicine, stress is laid on developing a person's immune system so that he is no longer susceptible to diseases. For the same reason, healthy food habits and nutritional guidelines are described in great detail in most *āyuṛvedic* texts[13].

♦ Role of dietary regimen and simple food

Great care is taken to prescribe diet which is in accordance with the body constitution and medical history of the patient. This hastens the healing process[14]. In contrast, diet that is not suitable for the constitution of the patient or might aggravate the problem, is prohibited. This dietary regimen strengthens the immune system in healthy people on one hand and on the other helps in quick recovery of the sick.

---

11. *Çhyawanprashaḥ : "Lehaṃ vaḥnibalaṃ ḍraṣṭavā khadeṭ*
kṣēenō rasāyanaṃ
Bāalvṛiḍh kṣatakṣēeṇā nārīkṣēeṇāṣçha śo ṣinaḥ"
ḥridoginaḥ ṣwarakṣēeṇā ye narāṣtēṣu yuçhyatē
kāsaṃ śwāasaṃ pipāsāṃ çha vāta ṣramuraśo grahaṃ
Vātapiṭtaṃ śukradōśaṃ mōoṭradośaṃ çha nāśayēṭ
Mēdhā ṣmritiṃ ṣtriṣu haṛṣaṃ kāṇti vaṛṇaprasaṇnatāaṃ
Aṣya ṗrayogādapṇoti narō jēeṛnavivaṛjitaḥ
(Sha. Ma.Kh. 8/19-20)

12. *Chanḍrapṛabhāvatti :*
"Çhanḍrapṛeti viḳhayātā saṛvarogpraṇāśiṇī
Ṗrēhāṇ viṇśati ḳriçheehūṃ mōotrāghātaṃ tathāṣmarēeṃ
vibaṇdhāssnāhaśōolāaṇī mehaṇaṃ graṇthimaṛbudaṃ
Āṇtravṛidhiṃ kaṭiśōolaṃ śwāasaṃ kāasaṃ viçhaṛchikāṃ
Aṇḍavridhiṃ tathā pāṇḍu kamlāṃ çha halēemakaṃ
Kuśṭhanyaṛśāsi kaṇduṃ çha pḷeehōdarabhagaṇdaraṃ
Daṇrōgaṃ nēṭrarōgaṃ ṣtrēeṇāmārtavajāṃ rūjaṃ
Puṇsāṃ śuḳragataṇ dośāṇ maṇdagnimaruçhiṃ tatha
Vāyu piṭtam kaghaṃ haṇyāḍ balyā vṛiśyā rasāyanī
Chanḍraprabhānāṃ kaṛṣaṣtu çhatuḥśāaṇō vidhīyatē
(Sha. ma Raj. 7/45-49)

13. *Āahāarasaṃbhavaṃ vaṣtu rogāṣçhāhārasaṃbhavāḥ* *(Ch.Su. 28/45)*

14. *Pōojayedaśanaṃ niṭyaḍyāaçhyāitadakuṭsayaṇ*
Ḍraśṭvā ḥriṇyēṭ praśeedēçhçha pratinaṇḍēçhya saṛvaśaḥ
Pōojitaṃ ḥyaśanaṃ niṭyaṃ balamōorjam çha yachhti
Apōojitaṃ tu taḍbhuḳtamubḥayaṃ nāśayēdidaṃ

♦ Simple and affordable remedies

In modern health care system, treatment does not even begin until several expensive tests have been carried out. This creates avoidable physical, mental and economical stress on the patient. In contrast, a good *āyuṛvedic* practitioner can diagnose the ailment merely by examining the patient's pulse etc. This helps to avoid unnecessary stress, delay and expenditure[15].

♦ Cure targets the root of the ailment

One of the unique features of this system of medicine is that treatment is aimed at eliminating the root cause of ailments and not by merely suppressing the symptoms. Elimination of the root cause ensures permanent cure.

♦ Conservation of ancient medical tradition

Practising *ayuṛved* ensures conservation of precious ancient knowledge gathered by our sages over the millenia. We thus contribute towards saving a time-tested and effective system of health care from the onslaught of instant but incomplete systems of medicine.

♦ *Ayuṛvedic* remedies: natural and easily available

Procuring most *āyuṛvedic* medicines is very easy, as numerous herbs are available in the kitchens and gardens. Another benefit of using *āyuṛvedic* medicines is that since one is using natural products, it keeps one in contact with nature and prevents one from being carried away by the modern technological and somewhat artificial life.

♦ Conserving foreign reserve

Keeping in view the economy of the country it is beneficial to use *Ayurvedic* medicines because These are available with in the country . Foreign exchange is spent to import expensive medicines from other countries. This unnecessary expenditure can be prevented if people start using medicines prepared in India. Conversely, the rising popularity of *āyuṛvedic* system of healing and medicines brings in precious foreign exchange.

---

15. *Darśanspaṛśan pṛaṣnāiḥ parēekṣeta c̣ha rōgiṇām*
Rōgaṃ nidānaṃ pṛagplakṣ́anōpśayāp̣tibhiḥ *(A.Saṃ.Su. 1/45)*

Rōgākṛānṭaḥ śarēeraṣya ṣthāanāaṇyaśṭāu pṛarēekṣ́yēṭ
Nāḍī mōoṭraṃ malaṃ jēeṿhā śaḅdaṃ ṣpaṛśa ḍrigākṛitiḥ *(Yoga. Ratnākar)*

Ṣaḍviḍhā hi rogāṇāṃ vigyanōpāyāaḥ - paṇchbhiḥ
śrōṭrādibhiḥ pṛaṣnēna c̣heti *(Su.Sū. 10/4)*

Taṣmādāturaṃ parēekṣ́ēṭ pṛakṛatitaśc̣ha
vikṛititaśc̣ha, sārataśc̣ha, saṇhananṭaśc̣ha, pṛamāṇataṣ́ c̣ha,
Sāṭṃyataśc̣ha, satvātaśc̣ha, āhāraśakṭitaśc̣ha,
vyāyāmaśatitaśc̣ha, vayaṣṭaṣ́cheti balapṛamāṇaviśeṣa
grahaṇa hetōḥ *(ch. Viman 8/94)*

♦ Complementary to *Yog* and *Dhaṛm*

As stated earlier, *Ayuṛved* provides complete knowledge on how to live a full and healthy life. It is thus very intricately bound with spirituality. Like life, it has its four goals:- the attainment of *Dhaṛm* (religion), *Arth* (benefit), *Kāam* (desire), and *Mokṣh* (Salvation)[16]. The principles and rules of *ayurved* help in the correct practice of *Yog*.

These characteristic features of *āyuṛvedic* healing system demonstrate that it is unique and different from other systems on account of being holistic and aiming at total well-being. Its greatest advantage is that it is in complete harmony with the natural rhythms of the human body.

3. Universal Status of *Āyuṛved*

Ayuṛved is concerned with the welfare of all living beings including plants and animals and not just humans. Together with treatises that enumerate various diseases afflicting human beings, there exist texts by different sages on the plant and animal diseases and their treatments. Amongst the better known are *Aśwayuṛved* (horse), *Gajāyuṛved* (elephant), *Gavayurved* (cow), and *Ṛrikśhāyurved* (tree).

The expertise and scope of *āyuṛved* is quite vast. On one hand it gives detailed information on how to treat rare and complex ailments (incurable) and on the other it teaches a healthy person to remain fit and disease-free[17,18]. Detailed and clear instructions about what to eat and when, what to avoid and how to conduct one's life are given in order to cultivate a healthy and stress-free lifestyle[19]. *Āyuṛved* also enumerates healthy and beneficial ways of attending to biological needs like hunger and thirst. It also describes how to deal with natural infirmities, i.e., the illnesses that accompany old age.

Eight general categories of topics in *āyuṛved*[20] There are :-

- ***Kāay Chikiṭsā*[21] :** Healing bodily

---

16. *Dhaṛmaṛthakāamamokśāṇāmārō gyaṃ mōolamuṭtamaṃ*
Rōgaṣtaṣyā ṗahaṛtāraḥ ṣ́rēyaso jēevitaṣya ċha

17. *Sāḍhyāsāḍhya vibhagagyō jgyānapōoṛvaka ċhikiṭsakaḥ*
Kāale ċhārabhatē kaṛm yaṭṭaṭ sāḍhayati ḍhruvaṃ *(Ch. Su. 10/7)*

18. *Ṗrayojanaṃ ċhaṣya (āyuṛvedaṣya) ṣwaṣthaṣya ṣwāṣthya rakśanaṃ* *(ch. Su. 30/26)*

19. *"Āahāar māṭrā ṗunarāgnibalāpekśiṇī"* *(ch. Su. 5/3)*
Ṛtāṿritāu ṇribhiḥ seṿyamaseṿyaṃ yaċhċha kiṇċhita
taṣyā śitēeyē niṛdiśṭaṃ hetumaṭsāṭmyamēva ċha *(ch. Su. 6/51)*

20. *Kāayavāalagrahoṛḍhvāṇgśaḷya bāal daṇśṭrā jarā ṿrisaiḥ*
Taḍyathā *(A.San. Sū. 1/10)*
Śalyaṃ, Śālāḳyaṃ, kāayċhikiṭsa, bhōotviḍyā,
Kāumāarabḥriṭyaṃ, agaḍataṇtra, rasāyāna taṇtra, vājīkaraṇ taṇṭramiti *(Su. Sū. 1/6)*

diseases through medication.

- ***Shalya Chikiṭsā***[22] **(Surgery):** Treatment by surgical intervention.
- ***Shaalakya Chikiṭsā***[23]**:** (7) This deals with problems of head, neck, eyes, ears, nose, mouth, throat etc.
- ***Agad Tantra*** **(Toxicology)**[24] **:** Deals with ailments caused by toxins.
- ***Bhōot Vidya*** **(Psychiatry) :** Treatment of mental disorders and psychiatric manegement.[25]
- ***Bāl Tantra*** **(Paediatrics)**[26] **:** Deals with illnesses of infants and children.
- ***Rasāyan Tantra*** **(Rejuvenation Therapy)**[27] **:** This branch of *Āyurved* deals with maintaining good health and minimizing the effects of old age infirmities.
- ***Vaajikaran Tantra*** **(Science of aphrodisiac)**[28] **:** Detailed treatment of low sperm count and similar problems.

A number of comprehensive treatises on all these categories were written by different sages and *āyuṛvedic* experts. Use of this highly effective medical system was common practice in the past but under hostile conditions during the Middle Ages, its practice was disrupted and declined. Several important texts

---

21. *Kāaya c̣hikiṭsānāṃ sarvāṇga sanṣ̣ritāanāaṃ vyadhēenāaṃ jwar, rakta, piṭta śoṣonmādapaṣmāar kuṣ̣thamehātisārādināmupṣamanāarthaṃ* (Su. Sū 1/3)
22. *Śalyaṃ nāama vividhaṭriṇakāaṣ̣thapāśāṇa pāṇśulōhalōṣ̣tāṣthi vālanakhapūyāṣrāvaduṇṭavṛiṇanṛgaṛbha Śalyāḍḍhaṛṇāartha yaṇtra, kṣāragni pṛaṇidhānavṛiṇa Viniṣ̣c̣hyaṛthaṣ̣c̣ha* (Su. Sū. 1/9)
23. *Śālākya nāamōṛdhvajatrugatāanāṃrogāṃ ṣ̣ravaṇanayana vadana ghrāṇādisaṇṣ̣ritānā vyadhināamupaśamanārthaṃ Śalākāyaṇtrapṛāṇīdhānārya* (Su. Sū 1/2)
24. *Agadataṇtraṃ nāam saṛpakēetalūtā mōośikādidaṇṭaviśavyajanāarth vividhaviśasaṇyogopaśamanāṛtha c̣ha* (Su. Sū. 1/14)
25. *Bhōotviḍya nāamadevāsuṛagaṇḍhaṛvayakṣarakṣapiṭripiśāc̣hanā gagrahāḍhupaṣriṣ̣tac̣hetasāṇ śāntikaṛmavali haṛṇādi grahopaśamanāṛthaṃ* (Su. Sū. 1/12)
26. *Kāumārabḥrityaṃ nāaṃ Kūmarabḥ araṇaḍhāṭrīkṣ̣ēeradośa saṇṣ̣ōḍhanāṛth duṣ̣ṭaṣṭaṇygrahasamutthānāṃ c̣ha Vyadhīnāmupaśamanāṛthaṃ* (Su. Sū. 1/13)
27. *Rasāyānataṇtraṃ nāam vayaḥ ṣthāyanamāyuṛmedhāvala Karaṃ rogāpaharaṇasamaṛthaṣ̣c̣ha* (Su. Sū. 1/15)
28. *Vājīkaraṇa taṇtra nāamalpaduṇṭakṣ̣ēeṇaviśuṣ̣karēṭa 5amāpyāyanapṛasādopac̣hayajonananiṃmitaṃpta haṛṣajananārthaṣ̣c̣ha* (Su. Sū. 1/16)

were either completely destroyed or lost. Paediatrics was perfected under the guidance of sage *Kashyap*. Sage *Sushrut* was a master surgeon. His '*Sushrut Saṃhita*' is easily available even today. Surgery was common and highly evolved. Caesarian operations and plastic surgery are described there in great detail. *Sushrut* had attained perfection in the art of plastic surgery. Complex procedures like *bhagaṇdar*, and removal of brain tumour were also performed. The popularity of surgery suffered a severe blow with the rise of Buddhism. In the backdrop of non-violence as propagated by Buddhism, surgery came to be regarded as a violent and painful practice and was hence given up. Other branches of *Āyuṛved* also suffered and today only the sciences of medicine, toxicology and aphrodisiacs are commonly practised. Other branches have all been lost.

Chapter 2

Fundamentals of *Āyuṛved*

1. The 5 elements and *Āyuṛved*

The four *Vedas* – *Rig*, *Saam*, *Yajuṛ* and *Athaṛv*- are considered to be the oldest texts and *Āyuṛved* originated from these ancient texts. It is considered a minor part of *Athaṛv ved*[29], although all four Vedas deal with different aspects of medicine and healing. In addition to describing all medicinal herbs and plants, the Vedas mention the basic principles *Doshas*[30] (*Vāyu*, *Piṭta*, *Kapha*), the seven *Dhātus* (*rasa*, *raḳta*,etc.), digestion and metabolism (*cyapcay*) processes. Other important principles of *āyuṛved* are also mentioned in the four Vedas. Thus the basic principles of *Āyuṛved* are in accordance with the honorable ancient Indian philosophical scriptures and text, in particular with *Śhaṇkhya Yog* and *Vaisheshik* schools of thought. Just as the *Sankhya* and *Yoga* texts believe that the five elements (air, water, fire, space and earth) combine to create the entire living and non living *(jad* and *chetan*) world, the fundamental belief of the *āyuṛved* is that the human body and its basic constituent elements and energy components – *Dosh*, *Dhātus* and *Mal* – are also made up of these five elements[31]. Although all basic elements are present in a substance, only one remains dominant. When the element of space dominates in a food item it is called *āakāśhiya*. Food products that have qualities of air are termed *vayavya diet*, the ones with water as the main constituents are *āapya diet* and the ones with predominance of earth element are termed *pāarthiv*. To identify what category an item belongs to, here is a brief description of the five categories:

♦ ***Āakāśhiya substances***: are soft, light, minute, plain. Eating of these increases softness, smallness, energy and pores in the body[32].

♦ ***Vayavya* Diet:** These food items are light, cool, rough, dry, sticky, minute and clear. Intake of these items increases roughness, hatred, speed, stickiness and

29. *Eh khalyāyaṛveda nāamupāṇgamathaṛava veda ṣyānu ṭpāḍēva pṛāgyāḥ* *(Su. Sū. 1/6)*
30. *Āahāaramagniḥ paçhati dośānāhāaravaṛjitaḥ dhātuṇ ḳśēeṇēsu dośēsu jēevitaṃ dhatu saṇḳśēya* *(A Wzi. chi 10/91)*
31. *Paṇçhabhōotāṭmā kē dēhē āhāraḥ pāṇchabhāutikaḥ Vipaḳvaḥ paṇchaḍha saṃyak guṇāna swāanabhi vaṛdhayēta* *(Su. Sū. 46/526)*
32. *Mridulaghusūḳṣmaślakṣana śabdaguṇna bahulāṇyākāśāaṭmakāani Tāni māaṛdavasāu ṣiṛyalāaghava karāaṇi* *(ch. Sū. 26/11)*

energy[33].

♦ ***Tejas* diet**: These are hot, pungent, minute, light, dry, non-sticky and cause beautifulness. Use of such foods increases burning, digestion, metabolism and lends healthy glow and complexion to the body. They also cause sensation of heat[34].

♦ ***Āapya* or *jalēey* diet:** These are liquid, cold, soft hard; moist and lend moisture and softness and increase determination and happiness[35].

♦ ***Pāarthiv* diet:** It is heavy, hard, non-sticky, thick, solid and odorous. These substances lead to an increase in the body weight and fat[36].

From the constituent elements of these diets and the constitution of the body, it is clear that the elements of Earth and Water predominate the body. The solid part of the body is made of Earth and the liquid part with Water. The empty spaces in the body are mostly the element of Space and very little part is Air[37]. The food we ingest is metabolized by the Fire element. In addition, various physical and mental processes are carried out with the help of the element of Air. The three *doshas*, (*vayu, pitta, kapha*) (*Ras, Rakt,* etc) the *dhātus* and the *malas* are also formed by the combination of the five basic elements. Different kinds of foods and medicines that nourish and treat the body are also constituted by these five elements. In food materials, the elements are identified by basic taste (*ras*), attributes (*guna*), potency (*virya*) and taste after digestion (*vipak*). Which element dominates which *dosha* - will be elaborated later. It is sufficient to note that whenever there is imbalance in the body, the diet that will either increase or decrease the affected element should be taken to restore harmony.

---

33. *Ślakṣạṇaṃ masṛiṇaṃ / ṿyavamēeti samaṣṭadēhaṃ ṿyāpta paśchāta pāakaṃ gaçhhati viṣamavadyavaṭi* (Dalhaṇ)
34. *Ūṣṇa tēekṣna sūkṣma laghu rōopaguṇa bahulāaṇyāagnēyāani Dahanaṃ bhaṣmasāṭkaṛnaṃ / pachanamāhārādipāa kaḥ Dāarṇaṃ ṿraṇāādēḥ / Pāatanaṃ śarēerādi Saṇṭāapanaṃ / Ṗrakāśanamabhi ṿyakṭiḥ / Ṗrabhā tējaḥ / vaṛnō Gāurāadiḥ* (Dalhaṇ)
35. *Śēetaṣṭibhitāaṣnigḍhamaṇda gurū sarasāṇḍra ṃridu picchilaṃ Rasbahulamēe ṣaṭkaṣāayāaṃlalavaṇaṃ madhuras ṗrāayamāa ṗyaṃ Baṇdhanaṃ parasparayoganaṃ / Ṗraḥlāadaḥ Śarēereṇḍriya taṛpanaṃl* (Su. Sū 41/5) (chakrapāaṇi)
36. *Taṭra ḍravyāaṇi gurukhara ḳathinamaṇdaṣthira viśadasāaṇḍra ṣthōola gaṇdha guṇabahulāahi pāaṛthivāani* (ch. Sū 26/11)
37. *Taṭra Vāyōrāaṭmāināaṭmāa, pittamāagnēyaṃ, ṣleṣmāa sāuṃya iti Vāayvāakāaśaḍhāātuḅhyāaṃ vāyuḥ, Āagnēyaṃpiṭṭaṃ Aṃbhaḥ ṗrithivēeḅhyāam ṣleṣmāa* (Su. Sū 42/5) (Aa. San. Sū 20/3)

2. The Principle of the 3 *Doshas*

Often when we consult an *āyuṛvedic* doctor or *vaidya* as they are known, they attribute our ailments to an increase in either *Vāyu, Piṭta* or *Kapha*. This normally leaves us confused because we have no idea what they are referring to. It's time we get acquainted with these terms[38].

Our bodies are made up of *doshas*, *dhātus* and *malas*[39]. All the constituent elements of our body are a part of these three, out of which, *doshas* are the most important on account of being the major constituents in the body.

There are three *Doshas:* 1. *Vāyu*, 2. *Piṭta* and 3. *Kapha*. Hence they are named tri-*doshas*[40]. It is these three *doshas* that are considered the pillars of the body and are responsible for its creation, preservation and destruction. Although it is the consummation of the sperm and ovum that gives birth to the body[41], without these *doshas*, the body cannot be formed. After birth, the nourishment of the body, maintenance of good health, prevention and cure of various ailments requires knowledge of the *tri doshas*. This is because all bodily processes – physical or chemical - are controlled by them. As long as these *doshas* are in their normal states and in balance, a person remains healthy. It is the imbalance in the normal levels of these *doshas* that results in ill-health[42]. The body becomes susceptible to disease. When the *doshas* are in balance, the *dhātus* and *malas*, and the elements that prevent ailments, are also in their normal states. But when the *doshas* lose balance it results in poor health and diseases. Because these *doshas*, due to an increase, decrease or dominance *(pṛakop)*, corrupt the essentially pure *dhātus* and *malas*, they are called *doshas* (literally translated, the word *dosha* means fault)[43].

There are two main reasons for the corruption of these *doshas*: (i) an increase in the levels present in the body and (ii) a decrease in the normal level. Most of the *mal* diseases are

---

38. *Sa aiva kupito dośaḥ samuṭthāana viśeṣataḥl*
Ṣthāanāaṇtaragataśçhāiva janayaṭ yāamayāana bahōoṇ
Tasmāaḍvikāara, pṛakṛitēeradhiṣṭhāaṇtarāaṇi çha
Samuṭthāana viśeṣāaṇṣçha baḍhhavāa Kaṛma samāachareta
Yo ḥyetat ṭritayaṃ jgyaṭvāa kaṛmamṇyāarabhateṭ bheṣaḳ *(Ch. Su. 18/45-47)*

39. *Dośadhāatu malamōolāṃ hi śarēeraṃ* *(Su.Su. 15/3)*
Dośadhatu malāamōolaṃ - Sadāa dehasya *(Aa. Hri. Su 11/1)*

40. *Vāyu pitfaṃ Kaphaśçhōḳtaḥ śāarēero dośasaṇgrahaḥ* *(Ch. Su. 1/51)*
Vāyu pitfaṃ Kaphaśçheti ṭrayodośāḥ samāasataḥ *(A. hr. Su. 1/6)*

41. *Śuḳraśōṇitaṃ gaṛbhaāśayaṣthamaātmapraḳriti vikaār*
Saṃmōoṛçḥitaṃ gaṛbh iṭyuçhyate *(Su. Sha 5/3)*

42. *Rogaṣtu dośa vāiśaṃyaṃ dośasāaṃyamāarogatāa* *(Aa. ḥri. Su 1/43)*

43. *Rasāadiṣthēṣu dośeṣu vyāaḍhayaḥ saṃbhavaṇti ye*
Tajjāaniṭyupçhāarēṇa tāanāahurḍhritadāahavaṭ *(Aa. ḥrisu. 1/32)*

caused by an increase in *dosha* because with a decrease in any *dosha*, its power to produce an illness is automatically reduced. It is true that with a reduction in the amount of a particular *dosha*, the contrasting element and attribute gains potency, and this again results in diseases related to the latter[44].

An increase in the amount of a *dosha*, corrupts the *dhātus* etc. and leads to ill-health. It is clear that a balance between the three *doshas* is absolutely essential. Only in a harmonious state can they work efficiently to maintain a healthy body[45].

Just as the mind permeates the entire body, so do the *doshas*[46]. The *doshas* are present even in such body parts and products as hair, nails and other body wastes. A brief introduction to the three *doshas* is as follows.

♦ *Vāyu* or *vāta*

This is the most important of the three *doshas*. The seed word of vata is 'va'. The elements that generate motion and vitality in the body constitute the *Vāyu dosha*[47]. *Vāyu* is the originator of all movements in the body. It governs all nervous functions, controls the mind, the senses and the motor organs. *Vāyu* is also responsible for the stimulation of the digestive juices and the enzymes that break down to digest food. The empty spaces of all the *srotas* in the body are also made of *Vāyu*. Composition of *Ras* (taste), blood and each *dhātu* (tissue elements), and the communication between various organs, are also due to the *Vāyu* element.

The foetus is nourished and develops in the womb due to *Vāyu*. It controls the entire nervous system. Without the *Vāyu dosha*, both the *Piṭta* and *Kapha doshas* become ineffective[48]. It is also responsible for the expulsion or excretion of urine and sweat from the body. When the *Vāyu dosha* is in a state of equilibrium, it keeps all *doshas*, *dhātus* and *malas* balanced. When it loses its balance and equilibrium, it corrupts other *doshas*, *dhātus*, and *malas*. Being active and mobile,

---

44. *Uṭkṛiśṭamaḍhyāalpatay¯tridhāa ṿridhi ķśyāavapi*
viķritāaśviķritāa dēhaṃ ghraṇti tē vaṛtayaṇti ḉha (A. San. Su 1/24)
Raśāadisṭhēṣu dōṣeṣu ṿyāaḍhayaḥ saṃbhavaṇti yē
Tajjāa niṭyapaḉhāarēṇa tāanāahuṛḍhritadāahavaṭ (A. San. 1/32)

45. *Samapiṭṭanilakaphaḥ kēchiḍgaṛbhāadi māaṇavāaḥ*
Ḍriśyaṃtē vāatalāaḥ kāaichiṭ piṭṭalāaḥ ślēṣmalāaṣtathāa
Tēṣāaṃanāaturāaḥ pōoṛvē vāatalāaḍyāaḥ sadāaturāaḥ
Dōśāanuśayitāa ḥyēṣāaṃ dēha pṛaķritiruḉhyatē (Ch. Su 7/39-40)

46. *Vāatapiṭṭaślē ṣmaṇāaṃ punaḥ saṛvaśarēera charāaṇāaṃ*
Saṛvāaṇiṣrōotāaṇṣyayana bhōotāani (Ch. Vi 5/6)
Vāatapiṭṭakaphāa dēhē saṛvaṣrōtosnusāariṇaḥ (Ch. Chi 28/59)

47. *Saṛvāa hi chēṣṭāa vāatēna sa pṛāaṇaḥ pṛāaṇināaṃ ṣmritaḥ*
Tēnāiva rōgāa jāayaṇtē tēna chāivōpāruḍhyatē (Ch. Su 17/118)

48. *Piṭtaṃ paṇgu kaghaḥ paṇguh paṇgavo malaḍhāatavaḥ*
Vāyuṇa yatra nēeyaṇtē taṭra gaḉhhaṇtimē ghavaṭ (Shāa. Pū 5/25)

the *Vāyu dosha* can transport other *doshas* to other parts of body where they are not required, increasing their levels and causing imbalances[49].

Hence it is clear that all ailments are due to the imbalance or corruption of the *Vāyu dosha*. When it is in balance, it maintains harmony among other *doshas*, *dhātus* and *malas*. When it is inflamed, it causes inappropriate mixing of these, which results in ill-health[50].

A very important characteristic of the *Vāyu dosha* is that it takes on the attributes of other *doshas* and this the cause of many diseases. When it interacts with *Piṭta doshas*, it takes on the characteristic of heat and on interaction with *Kapha* it becomes cold and moist[51]. *Vāyu dosha* has five divisions according to location and function. They are[52]

1. *Prāna* (life breath)
2. *Udāna* (rising air)
3. *Samana* (one of the 5 vital airs)
4. *Apāna* (downward breath)
5. *Vyāna* (diffused throughout the body)

The maladies caused only due to disturbances in the *Vāyu* are 80 in number.

◆ *Pitta*

Pitta constitutes the heat in the body. *Tapa* means heat or energy, so that which generates heat energy in the body, is called *Pitta*.[53] It regulates the enzymes and the hormones in the body. Whatever is ingested as food, and the oxygen we breathe-in, are converted to body elements (*doshas*, *dhātus*, *mala*) by the action of *Pitta*. Although *Pitta* and *Agni* (enzymes) are two different elements, it is *Pitta* that represents enzymes in the body. In other words, like enzymes, *pitta* maintains body temperature and digests food. It imparts colour to blood, skin etc., gives form and beauty to the body, keeps the heart healthy and absorbs oily substances that are massaged into skin and lends it glaze. In addition, *Pitta* also controls mental functions like intellect, valour, courage and happiness[54].

When *Pitta* is not in balance, the digestion is adversely affected. Energy levels go down and

---

49. *Sarvāa hi chēṣṭāa vāatēna sa prāṇaḥ prāaṇiṇāaṃ ṣmritaḥ*
    Tēnāiva rōgāa jāayatē tēna chāivoprōoḍhyatē   *(Ch.Sū-17/118)*

50. *Dośa ṭrayaṣya yasmāachha prakopē vāyurēeśvaraḥ*
    Vāta piṭta kaphā dēhē sarvaṣrotāa5nusāariṇaḥ
    Vāyurēva hi sūkṣmaṭvāada ḍwayoṣtatrāapyudēeraṇaḥ
    Kupitaṣṭāu samuḍdhōoya taṭra taṭra kṣipaṇ gadāaṇ   *(Ch. Chi-28/5960)*

51. *Yogavāha Paraṃ vāyuḥ saṇyōgāadubhayāaṛthakṛiṭ*
    Dāahaḳriṭ tējasāa yuḳtaḥ śeetakṛiṭ sōmasaṇśrayāaṭ   *(Ch. Chi-3/38)*
    Yogāaḍ yogino guṇaṃ vahtēeti Yogavāhaḥ
    Paramiti aṭyaṛtham   *(Chakrapani, Charak, Chi,ke.3rd Ch.)*

52. *Prāṇōdāanasamāanoavyāanāapāanāapāa nāiḥ sa panchadhāa*
    Dēhaṃ taṇtrayatē saṃyak ṣthāanēṣvavayāaḥṛitaścharaṇ   *(Ch. Chi. 28/5)*

53. *Pittaṣya dāaharāagōṣmapāakitāaḥ*   *(A.ḥri. Su 12/51)*
    Ūṣmāa pittāahatē nāasti   *(A.hri.Su. 1/16)*

Kapha begins to accumulate in heart and lungs. The five classes of *Pitta* are:[55]

1. *Pāchak Pitta* (digestive)
2. *Raṇjak Pitta* (bright red, colouring, gratifying etc.)
3. *Sāḍhak Pitta* (effective, efficient)
4. *Āalochak Pitta* (sight)
5. *Bhrajak Pitta* (sheen, glaze)

40 types of ailments are caused due to irregularities in *Pitta*.

Kapha or *Sleshma* (mucus)

Kapha means that which originates from water and *Sleshma* means that which joins and leads to cohesion.[56] This *dosha* provides nutrition to all parts of the body and regulates the two other *doshas*- *Pitta* and *Vāyu*. It makes the organs of the body moist and unctuous (oily, smooth and shiny) and lubricates the joints; increases libido, strength, enthusiasm, heals wounds, strengthens immunity, provides energy, and regulates patience, knowledge, wisdom, mental balance etc[57]. When there is an increase in heat due to *Pitta* or dryness due to *Vāyu*; *Kapha*, by increasing the quantity of oily and smooth fluids, protects the tissues from wear and tear. It is also the primary reason for sleep and lethargy/ inertia (*tāmas*). There is an increase in the body of *Pitta* and *Vāyu* when the amount of *Kapha* decreases. This results in damage of the *dhātus* (tissue-elements) by *Pitta* and accumulation of *Vāyu* in the *dhātus*, joints, heart and body parts. When *Kapha* is in balance, it nourishes the cells and body constituents.

The five types of *Kapha* according to location and function are:[58]

1. *Kledak* (that which moistens)
2. *Avalambak* (that which supports and energises)
3. *Bodhak* (that which lends and sharpens perception)
4. *Tarpak* (that which satisfies)
5. *Sleshak* (that which connects)

Doshas and the Five Elements

Like everything else, the *doshas* are also made up of the five elements. The predominant

---

54. *Taduḳtaṃ ḳrodhaśōkaṣ ram ḳritaḥ śarēerōṣmāa śirōgataḥ*
Pittaṃ ça keśāaṇ pachati palitaṃ tēna jāayatē (Su.Ni. 13-36)
Budhhimēdhabhimāanāaḍyāirabhipṛētāaṭth sāaḍhanāaṭ
Sāadhakaṇḥridagataṃ pittaṃ (A.hṛi.Su-12/13)
55. *Ataḥ paraṃ paṇchadhāa vibhajyaṇtē pitlaṣya*
Yaḳritapḷēehāanāuḥridayaṃ ḍriṣṭiṣṭwaḳ pōoṛvoḳtaṃcha (Sū.Sū-21/7)
56. *Kēna Jalēna niṇyaḍyatē cti kapha* (Sū. Sū. 21/7)
57. *Ṣnēhō baṇdhaḥ ṣthiraṭwaṃ ça gāuravaṃ vṛiśatāa balaṃ*
Ḳṣmāa ḍhritiralōmaṣçha kaphakaṛmavikāarajaṃ (Ch.Su. 18/51)
58. *Avalaṃbakaḳlēdakabodhakataṛpakṣḷeśakaṭvabhedāiḥ*
Ṣḷeṣmāa (A. San. Su. 20/6)

element in each *dosha* is as follows[59].

Dosha	**Predominant element**
Vāyu	Space and Air
Piṭta	Fire and Water
Kapha	Water and Earth

Doshas and Their Location In The Body

Although pervading the entire body, the *doshas* are prominent in certain organs and body parts[60].

Dosha	**Location**
Vāyu	Below the navel, urinary bladder, intestines, pelvic region, thighs,legs and bones.
Piṭta	Between navel and chest, sweat, lymph, blood and stomach
Kapha	Upper part of throat, head, neck, joints, upper portion of stomach and fat tissues of the body.

♦ *Doshas* and Seasons

The three *doshas* do not remain in balance constantly. All circumstances, favourable and unfavourable to any of the attributes of the *doshas*, affect them directly. They are also affected and transformed with the change in seasons, time of the day, condition of different body parts and psychological condition. Based on this, *doshas* have three conditions:

1. *Sanchay*: (accumulation).
2. *Prakop* (aggravation)
3. *Praśhman*[61]. (in normal batanced state)

It is recommended that to keep *doshas* in harmony, suitable diet according to the seasons must be taken.

Doshas and Agni (Digestive Enzymes)

Agni or digestive enzymes aid digestion and assimilation. This will be described later. Here it is important to mention that due to *doshas*, the intensity of *agni* also gets affected.

---

59. *Vāayvāakāaśaḍhātuḅhyāaṃ vāyuḥ Āagnēyaṃ piṭtaṃ*
Aṃbhaḥ p̣rithivēebḥyāaṃ śleṣmāah (A.San.Su-20/3)

60. *Taṭra paḳvāaśayaḥ kaṭiḥ saḳthinēe pāadāavāaṣthi*
Śroṭraṃ sparṣanaṃ c̣ha vāta ṣthāanāani
Aṭra c̣ha paḳvāaśay viśēṣvēṇa
Nāabhirāamāa śayaṣvēdō lasikāa rudhiraṃ c̣hakśuḥ
Sparśanaṃ c̣ha piṭta ṣthāanāani
Aṭra nāabhiṛviśeṣeṇa
Uraḥ kaṇthaḥ śiraḥ ḳlōma parvāaṇyāamāa śayo raso
medo ghrāaṇaṃ rasanaṃ c̣ha śeṣeṇa śleṣmaṣthāa nāani
Aṭrāapyurō viśēṣēṇa (A.San.Sū-20/3)

61. *C̣hayōṿriḍhiḥ ṣwadhāaṃnyēva pradvēso ṿridhi hetuṣu*
Vipreētaguṇeċhhāa c̣ha kopaṣṭōoṇmāargā gāamittāa (A. San. Sū. 20/9)

Dosha	**Intensity of *Agni***
Vāyu	Irregular
Piṭta	Intense (excessive)
Kapha	Slow (sluggish)
Vāyu, Piṭta, Kapha in equilibrium	Even Agni[62]

Doshas **and** ***Kośhth***

It has been documented that some people pass stool easily and require a very mild remedy (eg: a glass of milk) when they suffer from constipation. Others, under the same condition, require stronger remedies. There are some others who need very strong medication before

***Doshas*, Seasons and Time**[63]

S. No.	Name and Function of *Srota*	Controlling Organ (Origin)	Causes of Vitiation (Contamination)	Signs/Symptoms	Treatment
1.	*Prāna Vaha srota* (carrying vitality, vital breath)	Heart and alimentary tract	Wasting, suppression Of natural urges, intake of dry food, exercise when hungry	Long, restricted shallow & frequent Breathing. (Asthma is related to it)	Similar to breathing ailments
2.	*Udaka vaha srota* (carrying water, fluid part of body)	Palate, pancreas	Exposure to heat, indigestion, excess alcohol, intake of excessively dry food & excessive thirst	Dryness of palate, lips, tongue and throat	Treatment of thirst
3.	*Aṇna vaha srota* (carrying food taken from outside)	Stomach, left side of the body	Untimely food, overeating, unwholesome food and weak digestion	Loss of appetite (anorexia indigestion, vomiting)	Same as treatment for indigestion
4.	*Rasavaha srota* (carrying chyle, lymph, plasma)	Heart and ten vessels connected with heart	Worry & intake of excessively heavy and oily food	Anorexia, disgeusia, ageusia, nausea, heaviness, anaemia, impotency.	Fasting
5.	*Rakṭa vaha srota* (carrying blood especially the haemoglobin fraction)	Liver, spleen	Irritant, hot and oily food, excessive exposure to sun and fire	Serious skin diseases, bleeding, abscesses, inflammation in anus and genital organs	Blood-letting from related organ.
6.	*Māṃsa vaha srota* (carrying ingredients of muscle tissue)	Tendons, ligaments, skin	Sleeping immediately after meals, frequent intake of heavy and gross food	Granuloma, myeloma, uvulitis, goiter, adenitis, tonsillitis, many types of cancers and non-malignant growths	Surgical intervention etc.
7.	*Medo vaha srota*	Kidneys, abdominal fat and digestion	Lack of exercise, day time sleeping (suppresses enzymes) excessive fatty food, alcohol	Serious urinary disorders including diabetes	Eliminating causes

62. *Taṭra sama vātapiṭta śleṣamanāaṃ prakritiṣthanāanāaṃ samāa bhavaṇṭyagṇayaḥ*
Vāatalāanāaṃ tu vāatāabhibhāotē5gṇyadhiṣthāanē viṣamāa Dhavaṇṭyagṇayaḥ
Pittalāanāaṃ tu piṭṭāabhibhōotē hyagṇyadhiṣthāanē tēekṡnāaḥ bhavaṇṭyagnayaḥ
Śleṣmalāanāaṃ śleṣmāabhibhōotē5gṇyadhiṣthāanē maṇdāa bhavaṇṭyagnayaḥ (*Charak vimāan 6/12*)

they can feel relief. These three conditions are also connected with the *doshas*:[64]

Doshas	Kośhth (Stomach)
Vāyu	*Ḳrōor* (sluggish bowels)
Piṭta	*Ṃridu*
Kapha	*Maḍhyam* (moderate)
Vāyu, *Piṭta*, *Kapha* in balance	*Maḍhyam* (moderate)

The *doshas* are affected by external conditions and in turn affect all constituents and activities of the body. Their attributes are also affected by interaction with each other. Therefore, it is essential to know the attributes and behaviour of each *doshas*, and how different food items affect them, in order to keep them balanced and in harmony.

All three *doshas* are present in every person's body. But it is often one or two that dominate.The attributes of these dominant *doshas* dictate the body constitution and character of the person[65]. The physician thus, on examining the body and the character, is able to decide which *dosha*s is/are dominant and which are weak. This helps him to prescribe the proper remedy, diet and lifestyle change.Now we describe the nature and attributes of *Vayu Dosha*.

---

63. *Ṗraṭyōoṣaṣyaparāaạṇa ç̣ha jēerṇasṇhē ç̣ha ṗrakuṗyati* *(Su.Sū-21/20)*
Tataṭ varṣāaṣvōṣadhayaṣtarōoṇyō5lpavēeoṛyāa
. *āapaṣç̣hāapraśāaṇtāaḥ kṣ̣iti mataprāayāaḥ* *(Su.Sū 6/11)*
Taduṣ̣ṇāiruṣ̣ṇakāalē ç̣ha ghanāantē ç̣ha viśeṣatah
. *Maḍhyāaṇhē chāaṛdharāatrē ç̣ha jēeṛyaṇyaṇṇē ç̣ha kuṗyate* *(Su.Sū - 21/22)*
Tāa Aivāuṣadhayaḥ kāala pariṇāamāaṭ pariṇatavēeṛyāa
Valvaṭyō hemaṇta bhavaṇṭyaapaṣç̣ha praśāaṇtāḥ
. *Ṣnigdhāaḥ aṭyaṛtha guṛvgaṣcha* *(Su.Sū - 6/11)*
Sa Ścetācih sēetakāalē ç̣ha vasaṇtē ç̣ha viśēṣ̣ataḥ
. *Pōorvāaṇhē ç̣ha pradośu ç̣ha bhuktamaatrē ṗrakuṗyati* *(Su.Sū - 21/24)*

64. *Tāirbhavēḍviṣamaṣṭēekṣ̣nō maṇdaṣç̣hāagniḥ samaiḥ samaḥ*
Kośṭhaḥ ḳrōorō ṃriduṛmaḍhyō maḍhyaḥ ṣ̣yāatāiḥ samāirapi *(A.San.Sū 1/26)*
Tatra bahupiṭtō ṃriduḥ, Sa dugdhēnāapi viriç̣hyatē,
bahuvāataśḷeṣ̣māa ḳrōoraḥ, Sa duṛvirēç̣hya,
Samadośo maḍhyamaḥ sa sāadhāaraṇa iti. *(Su.chi 33/20)*

65. *Ṗrakritiḥ śuḳraśōṇitasaṇyōgē yō bhavēḍdośa uṭḳriṣ̣taḥ*
Ṗrakritiṛjāayatē tēna *(Su.Shā. 4/63)*
Kāalāadayaṣç̣ha śuḳraśōṇitamēva kuṛvaṇtaḥ praḳritijanakaḥ
bavaṇṭēeti taṇtrāaṇtarē śuḳraśohitagatadośenāiva
ṗraḳriṭyuṭṗāado daṛśitaḥ *(Ch.Vim. 8/95)*

3. *Vāyu* or *Vat Dosha*: Natural Attributes

Vāyu is dry, cold, light, minute, rough, clear and active. These are the natural attributes of *Vāyu*. When *Vāyu* is in balance, its attributes cannot be felt[66]. They can be experienced only during breathing or in a state of excitement. Qualities like dryness are manifested only when it gets aggravated.

	Attribute Effects/ Constitutional manifestations
1. *Rōokśh*[67] (dry, rough)	Dryness, emaciation and dwarfism of the body. Low, obstructed and hoarse voice and lack of sleep.
2. *Laghu*[68] (light)	Inconsistent gait, action, food and movement. Lightness in the body.
3. *Chanṇchal*[69] (mobile)	Unstable joints, eyes, eyebrows, jaws, lips, tongue, head, shoulder, hands and legs.
4. *Sheeghra* (swift)	Quick in initiating actions, *(ga- mita)* getting irritated, getting scared, catching diseases and infections, quickly deciding likes and dislikes, and swift in understanding and forgetfulness.
5. *Sheetal*[70] (cool)	Inability to bear cold, getting afflicted with cold, stiffness and shivering easily.
6. *Formaṭv*[71] (roughness)	Dry and rough hair, nails, teeth, face, hands and feet.
7. *Viśhdata*[72] (non-oily)	Dryness and cracked skin. Crackling sound on limb movement.
8. *Bahula* (abundance)	Talkativeness, abundance in tendons and veins.

66. *Tatra rōokśō laghuḥ śēetaḥ kharaḥ sūkṣmaṣchalo5nilaḥ* *(A.San.Su 1/28)*
Utsāahōçhwāasaniḥśwāasaçhēṣṭāa dhatugatiḥ samāa
Samō mokśō gatimatāaṃ vāayoḥ karmāavikāarajaṃ *(Ch.Su.18/49)*
Āaśukāarēe muhuṣ chāarēe paḳwāadhāan gudāalayaḥ
dehe vicharataṣṭaṣya lakṣnāani nibodh mē

67. *Yaṣya śoṣanē śaḳtiḥ sa rōokśaḥ* *(Hemadri)*
Rōokṣaṃ samēeraṇakaraṃ paraṃ kaphaghnaṃ mataṃ *(Bhāavaprakāaś)*

68. *Laghu Paṭhyaṃ paraṃ ṗroḳtaṃ kapuhanaṃ śēeghrapāakēp ça*
Laghuṣṣtaḍviṗrēetaḥ ṣyāalḷēkhanō ropaṇaṣtathāa *(Su.Sū - 46)*

♦ Symptoms Of Aggravated *Vāyu*

When *Vāyu* gets aggravated, it leads to dryness, roughness, stiff body and organs, pain similar to needle pricks, loosening of joints, displacement of bones, brittle bones, hardness, weak organs, shivering and swift numbness in limbs, feeling cold, weakness, constipation, *shool* (pain in nails and teeth, discoloration and dull skin, losing taste etc).[73]

Vāyu gets aggravated and affects the intestines. When waste (*mala*) food reaches the intestines, aggravated *Vāyu* is generated.

♦ Reasons for Aggravation

Suppressing natural urges like excretion, urination, sneezing, eating before digestion of previous meal, sleeping late, talking loudly, working more than ones capacity, bumpy ride in vehicles, eating too much dry, pungent, bitter and astringent foods, overeating dryfruits, worrying and being tense constantly, overindulgence in sexual activity, fasting, overeating, eating cold food and being afraid – all these conditions aggravate *Vāyu*. In people with *Vāyu* constitutions, even minor causes will often lead to *Vāyu* aggravation.[74]

♦ Treatment of Aggravated *Vāyu*

To restore balance of *Vāyu*, the causes of aggravation have to be ascertained followed by intake of food and medication that will counter the reasons for the same. In addition,

---

69. *Yaṣya Pṛēraṇē śakti sa sarah* (Hemadri)
Saraṣṭēśāam pravaṛtakaḥ (Bhāavaprakāsh)

70. *Staṃbhanē himaḥ* (hemadri)
ḥwāadanaḥ ṣtaṃbhanaḥ śēetō mōoṛchhāatṛitṣwēdadāahajit. (Su.Sū - 46)

71. *Yasya lekhanē śaktiḥ sa kharaḥ* (hemadri)
Kaṛkaṣtwam vāayavyaḥ (R.vā.A.2, Sū 60)

72. *Yaṣya kṣāalanē śaktiḥsa viśadaḥ* (hemadri)
Viśadō viprēetō5ṣmāaṭ kḷedāachōo Ṣaṇarōpaṇaḥ (Su.Sū 46)
Kḷedachhēdakaraḥ ḳhyāatō viśsadō vṛnaropaṇaḥ (Bhāavprakash)

73. *Kāarśyakāarśuyogāatrakampasphuraṇanōṇa kāamitāa*
Saṇgyāanidṛāanāaśabalēṇdriyōpḍyāatāaṣthi śōolamajjaaśōṣamala
Saṇgadhmāanāaṭōpamōhadāiṇyabhayaśōkapralāapāadibhirvṛuḍhō
Vāyuḥ pēedayati (A.hr.Su. 11/6)
Saṇkoṭchaḥ paṛvanāaṃ ṣtaṃbhō bhēdō5ṣthnāaṃ paṛvanāamapi
Lōmaharṣa pralāapaśḉha pāaṇipriśṭh śirōgrahaḥ
Khaṇgya pāadāadāaṇulyaḥ kubjaṭwaṃ śōṣō5ngāanāaṃ niḍratāa (Ch.Chi. 28/20-21)

74. *Vēga saṇdhāaraṇāadāa māadabhighāatāada bhōjanāaṭ* (Ch. Chi. 28/17)
Taṭra balwadvigrahāativyayamavyavādhayana pṛapatanapra
dhāavanapra pēedanāabhighāataplawana taraṇarāatrī
jāagaraṇbhāaraharaṇna.... (Su.Sū - 21/19)
Taṭra vātalaṣya vātaprakopṇāanyāasēvmāanasya kṣipraṃ
Vātaḥ prakogamāapaḍyatē, na tathētarāu dośāu (Ch. Vim. 6/16)

treatment should be done keeping in mind the attributes of the *Vāyu dosha*. Following are the remedies for aggravated *Vāyu*[75] :

1. Consumption of oily substances (*ghēe*, oil, fats, *Piṭta*), bathing with warm water and enema.
2. Fomentation (induced sweating). Bathing or ingesting heat producing foods leading to sweating.
3. Mild purgation using medicines prepared from oily, hot, sweet, sour and salty substances in order to expel waste products.
4. Tying diseased organ with cloth and *pultis* (healing through medicated cloth) pressing them with hands and feet, massaging and bathing with *Vāyu* destroying substances and inhaling them.
5. Gently pouring *Vāyu*-controlling concoctions on the head.
6. Drinking medicated alcoholic preparations from *Vāyu*-controlling herbs and substances.
7. Using oil, *ghēe* and other oily foods medicated with *Vāyu*-decreasing and purgative herbal medicines.
8. Eating food containing wheat and jaggery.
9. Various types of enema using herbal medicines made from hot and oily substances.
10. Psychological treatment according to ailment and the condition of the patient.

Oil is the most important of all *Vāyu*-pacifying oleac substances[76]. Sesame oil, fat-rich meat, the juices of such meat for non-vegetarians and *anuvāsana* (a type of enema) are particularly beneficial for patients with vitiated *Vāyu*. As the primary location of *Vāyu* in the body is the large intestine, *niruh* and *anuvāsana* enema are the best cures for this. Medicated substances are introduced through the rectum for easy and fast expulsion of impurities from the body and restoration of balance of the *Vāyu dosha* by directing the treatment to the source of the trouble[77].

---

75. *Rōokṣaḥ śēetō laghuḥ sukṣmaśçhalo5th viśadaḥ kharaḥ*
Viprēetaguṇāiṛḍravyāṛmāarūtāḥ saṃpraśāaṃyati *(Ch.Sū -1/59)*

76. *Tilapṛiyāalāakṣodāadayō5nēkāa yōnayō yēṣāaṃ tē5nēkayonyaḥ ṣnehāa* *(A. San. Su. 13/3, Armdatta)*
Māarutaghnaṃ na çha śkṣmavaṛdhanaṃ balvaṃdhanaṃ
Twaçhyamuṣṇaṃ ṣthiṛakarṃ tailaṃ yōniviśodhanaṃ *(Ch. Su. 13/15)*
Taḍvaṣṭiṣu çha pāanēṣu naṣyē karṇāakṣi pōoraṇē
Aṇnapāanavidhāu chāapi ṗrayoj̣yaṃ vātāśāanṭayē *(Su. Sū. 45/113)*
Ya ṣnehāiṛdēeyatē Saḥ ṣyāadanuvāasananāamakaḥ
Kaṣāaya kṣēeratāilāiṛyō nirōohaḥ sa nigaḍyate *(Sha. U. 575)*
Anuvāaṣyaṣtu rookśaḥ ṣyāaṭṭēekṣna gniḥ kevalāanileeh *(Sha. U. 515)*
Vāatavỵāadhāavudāavaṛtē vāatāaṣrigviṣamajwarē
Mōorçhḥāaṭrīṣṇōdarāanāahamōoṭra kṛuçhhāaśmarēeṣu çha
Ṿridhāaṣrigdaramaṇdagniprамēhēṣu nirūharaṇaṃ
Sōole5mla pittēḥriḍrōgē yōjayēḍvidhivaḍ budhaḥ *(Sha. U. Kha. 6/6-7)*

♦ Symptoms of Low *Vāyu* and Its Remedies

When the levels of *Vāyu* drop, there is a slowing down of various physiological functions, dipping of spirit (unhappiness), reduction in perceptive powers,weariness, disinterest in speech, slowing down of normal *Vāyu* functions and *kaphaj* (ailments caused due to *Kapha dosha* like indigestion, nausea etc.)[78]

To strengthen *Vāyu*, take food items that help to increase it. Light, cold, bitter, pungent and spicy foods increase *Vāyu*. In addition to these, food items listed under reasons for aggravation of *Vāyu*, must be consumed[79].

♦ *Sāam* and *Nirāam Vāyu*

When *Vāyu* mixes with *āam-ras* (accumulated undigested part of food in the body) it is called *Sāam*. The following symptoms are manifested in case of *Sāam* formation.

* Obstruction in expulsion of excreta, urine and *apāna Vāyu.*
* Weak digestion
* Laziness
* Intestinal disturbance
* Backache
* Rheumatism, arthritis and swelling of joints
* Pain similar to needle pricks[80]

If *Sāam vāyu* is not treated in the initial stages, it becomes vitiated and spreads throughout the body.

---

77. *Vāatanikāarāaḥ praśāṃtimāapadyanṭē, yathāa vanaspatērmōolē Çhhinnē ṣkanḍhaśāakhāa prarōhakusumphala palāaśadēenāaṃ niyatō uināaśaṣtadvaṭ* *(Charak Sut. 20/13)*

78. *Tatra, vāatkṣayē manḍacheṣṭatāa5lpavāakṭwamapraharṣō mōoḍhsangyṭāa cha* *(Su. Sū. - 15/11)*
Prasēkāaruchihrilḷāasaṣangyāmōhalpa vāaḳ
Chēṣtatāa praharṣāangi sāadāagni vāiṣaṃyāadibhiḥ kśēeṇō
Vāyuḥ pēeḍayati *(A. San. Su. 21/9)*
Lingaṃ kṣēeṇē5nilē5angaṣya sāadō5lpaṃ bhāaṣitēhitaṃ
Sangyamohaṣtatha śleṣmavriḍḍhyukṭāamaya saṃbhavaḥ *(A hri. Su. 11/15)*

79. *Tatra (Vāatakśayē) ṣwagōnivarḍhanāaṇyēva pratēekāaraḥ*
Vāatakṣayē kaṭutikṭakaṣāayarōokśalaghuśēetāanāaṃ *(Su. Sū. 15/12)*

80. *Sarva ḥa māarūtaṃ tanḍrāaṣtāimiṭyagāuravāiḥ*
Ṣnighaṭwarōçhakāalaṣyaśāityaśōphāagnihāanibhiḥ
Kaṭu rōokṣāabhilāaṣēṇa taḍvighōpaśayāyēna cha
Yukṭaṃ vidyāaṇnirāamaṃ tu tanḍradēenāaṃ viparyayāaṭ *(A. hri. Ni. 16/29-30)*
Vāyu Sāamō vivanḍhāagniṣaadāatanḍranṭra kōojanāiḥ
Vēdanāa śōphāniṣtodaiḥ kramaśo5ngāani pēe5yan
Vicharēḍhu gapacchāapi grahalāati kupito bhriśaṃ
Ṣnōhāadyaīrvridhimāapnōti suryamēdōdayē niśi *(A. hri. Su. 13/27)*

When *āam* is absent from *Vāyu*, it is called *Nirāam Vāyu* which causes dryness in the organ, mouth and tongue. and mild discomfort It should be treated by an unctuous (oily) diet[81].

♦ *Vāyu* and Its Division

Vāyu has been divided into five types based on its location and function. Each type is responsible for different ailments. The following table lists location, function and ailments.

Types of *Vāyu* and Their Functions

S.No.	Type	Location	Function	Illnesses due to vitiation
1.	*Prāṇa*[82] (Life breath)	Head, tongue, heart, throat, face and nose	Breathing and swallowing of food, conversion of breath into life force, spitting, sneezing, etc.	Hiccup, cough, asthma, cold and bad throat.
2.	*Udāna*[83] (Rising air)	Throat, navel, diaphragm, chest	Speech and voice, upward movement of breath, responsible for strength, enthusiasm and will to work	ENT and eye ailments
3.	*Samāna*[84] (Balancing air)	Stomach and intestinal tract	Stimulating gastric juices to break down food and categorizing them into *dhātus* and *malas*, digestion, assimilation, controlling *sved vaha jal vaha* and *dosh vaha srotas* (channels)	Weakness of digestive powers, indigestion, diarrhoea and defective assimilation
4.	*Apāna*[85] (downward and outward breath)	Large intestine, organs of the pelvicregion (kidneys, bladder, navel, rectum, etc.)	Expulsion of stool, urine, semen and menstrual fluid. Keeps foetus in place and helps during birth.	Diseases of bladder, anus, testicles, uterus and obstinate urinary ailments including diabetes.
5.	*Vyāna*[86] (outward moving air)	Entire body especially heart	Causes sweating, bending, getting up, movement of eyelids, yawning, helps in functioning of circulation channels, transports nourishing juices & blood through body.	Fever, diarrhoea, slowing down in the transmission function of srotas, bleeding and consumption.

---

81. *Niāamō viśadō rọokṣo nirvivaṇdho5lpavēdēvaḥ*
Viparēeta guṇāiḥ śāaṇti ṣnighāiṛyāati viśeṣataḥ (A.hri. Su. 13/28)

82. *Ṣtāanaṃ p̣rāṇaṣya mōoṛdhōraḥ kaṇthaṇ kaṛna Jiṿhaṣyanāasikāaḥ*
Ṣthēvanakṣ́vathōogāara śwāasāahāarāadi kaṛm c̣ha (Ch. Chi. 28/6)

4. Piṭta

In the three *doshas, Piṭta* comes next to *Vāyu*.

♦ Attributes

Piṭta is hot, slightly unctuous (greasy), pungent, liquid, swift and smells of flesh[87]. When it is in *nirāam* state, it is bitter in taste and yellow in colour. In the *sāam* state, it is sour and blue[88].

♦ Attributes Of *Piṭta* and Their Effects Of Physiology

Like *Vāyu*, *Piṭta* also helps to build the body and determine its nature. The various attributes of *Piṭta* and their effects on the body are listed in the following table:

---

83. *Udāanaṣya punaḥ ṣṭāanaṃ nāabhyuraḥ kaṇtha aiva ċha*
Vāaka pṛaṿrittiḥ pṛayan̄orjobalavaṛṇāadi kaṛm ċha (Ch. Chi. 28/7)
Udāanonāama Yaṣṭōoṛdhwamupāiti pawanōttamaḥ
Tēna bhāaṣilāgēetāadiviśēṣō5bhipravaṛtatē
Ūṛdhwajaṭru gatāaṇ rōgāaṇ karōti ċha viśeṣataḥ (Su. Ni. 1/14/15)

84. *Āamapaḳwāaśayaċharaḥ samāanōnaṇhisaṇhisaṇgataḥ*
5ōśṇnaṃ paohati tajjāaṇṣ̌cha viśeśāaṇvivinaḳtini
Gulṃāagni sāadāatēesāara pṛabhritēeṇ kurutē gadāaṇ (S.N. 1/16/17)
Swēdadōśāaṃbuvāahēeni ṣrōtāasi samadhiṣ́ṭiṭaḥ
Aṇtaragnēṣ̌cha pāaṛṣ̌vaṣ́thaḥ samāanōśgnibalapradaḥ (Ch. Chi 28/8)

85. *Ṿriśaṇān vaṣti mēḍraṃcha naaphyōoru vaṇḳṣ̌nān gudaṃ*
Apāanāṣthāanamaṇtraṣthaḥ śuḳramōotra śaḳriṇticha
Ṣrijaṭyāaṛtanagabtaān cha, yuḳtāaḥ ṣṭhāan ṣṭhitāaṣ̌cha te
Ṣwakaṛma kuṛvatē dēhō dhāaṛyatē tāiṛa nāamayaṇ (Ch. Chi 28/10-11)
Paḳwāadhāanāalayōśpāanali kāalākaṛṣaticháapyaṃ
Samēeraṇaḥ śaḳriṇmōotraṃ śuḳragaṛbhāaṛtavāanyadhaḥ ċha
Ḳruḍdjaṣcha kurute rōgāaṇ ghōrāaṇ vaṣti gudāaśṛayeiaṇ (Su. Ni. 1/19-20)

86. *Ḳriṭṣnadēhacharō Ṿyāanō rasasṇvahanōḍyataḥ*
Ṣwēdāa ṣrikṣrāa vaṇa ṣ̌ċhōo pi paṇchadhāa cheṣṭayaṭyapi
Ḳruḍdhaṣ̌cha karutē rōogāaṇ pṛāayaśaḥ sarvadēnagāaṇ (Su. Ni. 1/17/18)
Dēhaṃ vyāapṇōti sarvatuvyāanaḥ śēeghragatiṛṇriṇāaṃ
Gati pṛasāaraṇāapēḳṣapanimēṣāadikriyaṇ sadāa (cu. Chi 28/9)

87. *Saṣnēhamuṣṇaṃ tēekṣnaṃ ċha ḍravamamlaṃ saraṃ kaṭu*
Vipaṛēetaguṇāiḥ piṭtaṃ ḍravyāirāaśu pṛaśāaṃyati (Ch.Su. 1/60)
Kaṭivati tiḳtam pēetaṃ (Gangadhar)
Piṭtaṃ tēekṣ̌naṃ ḍravaṃ pōoti nēelaṃ pēetaṃ tathaiva ċha
Uśṇaṃ kaṭurasaṃ chāiva vidagdhaṃ chāamlamēva ċha (Su. Sū 21/11)

88. *Piṭtaṃ hi vidaṭgdhmamlatāamupāityāagniyaṭwāaṭ* (Su. Sū 42/10)
Mādhuryamaṇaaṃ gatamāanasaṇgyaṃ nidaghhasaṇgya
gatamaṃlabhāvaṃ, kiṇċhiḍ vipaṃvaṃ (Su. S̄ 46/509)

Attributes	Effects
1. *Uṣṭṇa*[89]	Intolerance for heat and hot things, having hot face, tender and clear body, heat freckles, black moles, excessive hunger and thirst, quick advent of wrinkles, greying of hair and baldness, soft, brown facial and body hair.
2. *Tikshnata*[90] (sharpness)	Tendency to demonstrate body strength, sharpness of character, strong digestive power, intake of food and drink in large quantity, gluttony, inability to face difficult situations.
3. *Dṛavata*[91] (liquid)	Tenderness and looseness of joints and muscles, sweating, urine and excreta in large quantity.
4. *Visragandnita*[92] (fleshy smell)	Strong odour in underarms, mouth, head and other body parts.
5. *Katu* and *Āmlā*[93] (Pungent and sour taste)	Low semen quantity, sexual desire and procreation ability.

When the *Piṭta dosha* dominates in the body, one is said to have a *Piṭta* constitution. The above mentioned properties of *Piṭta* result in moderate strength, life-span, material and spiritual knowledge, material assets etc[94].

♦ Symptoms of Aggravated *Piṭta*

Excessive *Piṭta* in the body leads to fatigue, lack of strength and sleep, excessive sweating, increased body temperature and burning sensation, darkening of complexion, body odour, stickiness, anger, dizziness and fainting, etc. Yellowing of skin, stool, urine, nails and eyes are unique symptoms of aggravated *Piṭta*. Craving for cold food and drink, and bitter/ sour taste in the mouth are also a result of heightened *Piṭta* levels in the body[95].

---

89. *Piṭtaṃ vaḥnirvaḥnijaṃ vāa padaṣmāaṭ pittoḍrikatạ*
Ṣwāarkṣ̣ṇaṭriṣ̣ṇāavṛimakṣ́aḥ
Gāurōṣ̣ṇāaṇgaṣṭāaṃrahaṣṭāaṇghri vakṭraḥ śurō māani piṇgkēśō5lparōma
90. *Dayita māalayavilēpaṣ̣maṇdanaḥ suçharita śuçhirāaṣritavatsalāaḥ*
Vibhavsāahasa budhibalāaṇvitō bhavati bhēeṣu śatidviṣāatāamapi
91. *Medhāavēe pṛaśethēela saṇdhivaṇdhamaṃsō nāarēenāamanamito5lpaśukṛamaṃsaḥ*
Āavāasaḥ palilataraṇgnēelikāanāaṃ madhur kaṣāayāatiktaśeetaṃ
92. *Dharṃdṿeṣēe ṣwēdanaḥ pōotigaṇdhirbharyōoçchāarakṛodhpāanāaśanērśyaḥ*
93. *Tanani piṇgāani çhalāani çhāiṣāṃ taṇvalpapakṣ̣māaṇi himpṛiyāaṇni* (A. hri. Sha. 3/10-14)
Ḳrodhēna maghēna śwēṣ̣çha bhāasāa rogaṃ varjaṇtyāaśu vilōçhanāani

♦ Causes

Consumption of large quantities of bitter, sour, hot, spicy, fermented food and drinks increases *Piṭta dosha* in the body. In addition, consuming dry vegetables and alkaline foods, too much exposure to heat and sun, excessive sexual intercourse, irregular food habits (not eating at fixed time, not eating when hungry, eating without hunger etc.), indigestion, anger, fear,depression etc. also affect the *Piṭta dosha*. Some food items like sesame oil, mustard, green vegetables, yoghurt, butter milk, cream of boiled milk, vinegar, intoxicating drinks, mutton etc. aggravate *Piṭta*[96].

♦ Remedies For Vitiated *Piṭta*

First the causes for aggravation of *Piṭta* must be addressed. *Virechan* (induced vomiting) is the best therapy[97]. *Piṭta* normally accumulates in the stomach and duodenum and the herbal preparation reaches these sites and clears out the *piṭta*.

Continuous intake of *ghēe* (clarified butter), which has opposing attributes like sweetness and coldness, is very useful. In fact long term *Piṭta* diseases are treated using different types of *ghēe*[98].

♦ Symptoms of Low *Piṭta* and Its Remedies

When the level of *Piṭta* falls in the body, there is a reduction in the digestive powers, body temperature, radiance, sheen on skin, and an increased awareness of cold. There is also a slowing down of the body processes controlled by *Piṭta*[99].

---

94. *Madhyāayaṣo madhyabalāah paṇḍitḥ kḷeśabhēeravaḥ*
Ṿyāaghrarkṣkapimāarjāarayakṣāanōokāaṣḉha pāittikāḥ

95. *Piṭtaṣya dāaharāagōśyapāakitāaḥ*
Ṣwedaḥ kḷedaḥ sṭrutiḥ kothaḥ sadanaṃ mōorcehanaṃ madeḥ (A.hri. Su. 12/41-42)
Katukāamlān raso varṇaḥ pāaṇḍurāaruṇa vaṛjitaḥ
Uśma piṭtadvattē nāaṣti (A.hri. Ch. 1/16)

96. *Krodha śōkabhayāasōpavāasavidagdha māithunōpagamana*
Katavaṃlalavaṇa tēekṣṇōṣṇaṃlaghuvidāahitilataila
pivyāakakulaṭtha saṛṣapāataseēharitakaśāakagōdhāamaṭṣyāa jāavikamāaṃ
Sadadhitakṛakōorchikāamaṣtu sāuvēerakaḥ surāavikāarāaṃla
phalakaṭvara pṛaḅhritibhiḥ piṭtaṃ pṛakopmāapadyatē (Su. Sū. - 21/21)

97. *Virēchan Piṭtam harāaṇāaṃ* (Ch. Sū. - 25/40)

98. *Kaṭwamvalavaṇāaḥ piṭtam* (Ch.Sū. -1/67)
Kaṣāaya ṣwāadutiḳtakāḥ Jayanti piṭtaṃ (Ch. Sū. 1/66)
Madhurtiḳta kaṣāayāaḥ piṭtaghnāḥ
Kaṭwamla lavaṇāaḥ piṭtaṃ janayantiḥ
Madhurtiktakaṣāayāaṣṭvēnaḉhhamayaṇti (Ch.Vim 1/6)
Ṣtambh śāitayāa miyatatōdadāahāarōchakāavipāakāaṇga
-pāarōonyakaṃpgāuravanakhanayana śāukḷyadibhiḥ piṭtaṃ (A. San, Su. 11/16)

99. *Piṭtakṣayē maṇḍōmāagnitāa niśprabhatwaṃ·ḉha* (Su. Sū. 15/11)
Pittē kṣēeṇē maṇḍō5nalaḥ śēetaṃ pṛabhāahāaniḥ (A.H.Su. 11/16)

In this condition, a regular intake of *Piṭta* increasing foods and medicines is useful, especially those that have the fire element in dominance. Similarly herbal preparations which increase fire or are rich in fire elements should be administered.

♦ *Sāam* And *Nirāam Piṭta*

When *Piṭta* mixes with *āam*, it turns fetid (stinks) and changes into a foul-smelling, oily, sour, heavy blackish green liquid. In this condition, sour eructation (belch) and heart-burning sensation in throat and chest are experienced[100].

When *Piṭta* is without *āam*, it is hot, odorous, bitter, red or yellow in colour, and mixes easily with water. It increases hunger and digestion.

On suffering from *Sāam Piṭta* i.e. *Piṭta with āam,* foods with bitter and pungent taste should be consumed. On the other hand, when suffering from *Nirāam Piṭta*, sweet and astringent foods should be ingested[101].

♦ Types of *Piṭta*

On the basis of location and function, *Piṭta* is divided into five categories mentioned below:

Piṭta And Its Divisions:[102]

S.No.	Type	Location	Function	Illnesses due to vitiation
1.	*Pāchak* (Dissolvent, digestive)	Stomach and central part of small intestine	Digestion, separation of nutrients and wastes after digestion, nourishing, other *Piṭta* locations and rest of the body with, heat generation, hunger and cravings	Indigestion
2.	*Ranjak* (lending colour)	Liver, spleen and stomach	Blood formation from the digested food energy	Anaemia, Jaundice etc.
3.	*Sāḍhak* (effective and efficient)	Heart	Cleansing the heart of dark thoughts and desires, increase intelligence, memory, wisdom and pride	Psychological disturbances, fear, anger, greed etc.
4.	*Ālochak* (vision)	Eyes	Lends vision	Impairment of vision
5.	*Bhrajak* (lustre shine)	Skin	Lending colour and lustre to skin, absorbing oily substances to nourish various body parts, maintaining natural heat of the body.	Leucoderma and other skin diseases

100. *Durgaṇdhi haritaṃ śyāavaṃ piṭtamaglaṃ dhanaṃ guru*
Amlēekāakaṇthahacchāahajaraṃ sāayaṃ viniṛdiśēṭ

101. *Āatāaṃrapatimatyuśṇaṃ rasē kaṭukamaṣthiraṃ*
Pakvaṃ vigaṇdhi vigyēya ruchipakṭibalapradaṃ (A.H. Su. 13/27/28 Middle)

5. *Kapha* or *Sleshma*

In order of importance, *Kapha dosha* is placed last. Following is the description of its various aspects.

♦ Attributes of *Kapha*

Kapha is oily, sweet, heavy, soft, firm, sticky, slow, cold, moist and white[103].

People with dominant *Kapha dosha* have *Kapha* body type. The following effects of *Kapha* manifest themselves in *Kapha* constitutions[104].

People with *Kapha* constitution have abundance of strength, material wealth,

	Attributes	Effects
1.	*Snigdha* (unctuous)	Unctuousness of organs
2.	*Sleksh* (smooth)	Smoothness of organs
3.	*Mṛidu* (soft)	Pleasing appearance, tenderness and clarity of complexion
4.	*Maḍhur* (sweet)	Increase in quantity of semen, libido and reproductive power
5.	*Dṛidta* (firm)	Compactness, strength and firmness of body
6.	*Ghaṇta*	Plumpness & rounded-ness of organs
7.	*Māṇd* (slow)	Slow in action, intake of food and movement
8.	*Sthirta* (firm)	Slowness in initiating actions, irritation, slow manifestation of serious illnesses.
9.	*Gurūta* (heavy)	Firm and steady gait entire sole touching the ground
10.	*Sheetalta* (cold)	Lack of intensity of hunger and thirst, low perspiration and not feeling heat.
11.	*Piçhchilta* (viscous)	Firmness and in joints

---

102. *Rāagapaḳti tējōmēdhōṣmaḳrit piṭtaṃ paṇchadhāa*
p̣ravidhaḳtamagni kaṛamaṇāa5nug̣rahaṃ karōti
Yaḍḍriṣṭyāaṃ piṭtaṃ taṣminṇāalōchakōgniriti sangyāa
sa ropag̣rahaṇāadhiḳritaḥ
Yaṭtu ṭwachi piṭtam taṣmiṇ ḅhrāajako5gniriti saṇgyāa
sō5ḅhyaṇgapariṣ̣ēkāavagāahāalē panāadēenāaṃ ḳriyāavṛavỵāaṇāaṃ
paḳtāa, chhaāanaaṃ ç̣ha p̣rakāaśakaḥ (Su Sū 21/10)
Vāata piṭta kapha vāyusūṛya ç̣haṇdra rōop hāi
sōma āiva śarēerā śḷēṣ̣māaṇtargataḥ kapiṭāakupitaḥ śubhāaśubhaani karōti (Ch. Su.12/12)

knowledge, and peace. They also have a long life-span[105].

♦ Symptoms of Vitiated *Kapha*

With an increase in the *kapha dosha* the following symptoms are manifested.

Feeling languid, increased sleep, sweet taste in the mouth, skin loses colour, feeling cold, itchy, heavy, stickiness of *mala* (body wastes like excreta, urine, sweat, etc.), a feeling of being wrapped in wet cloth, being covered with some substance, swelling, congestion, increased secretion of eye and nose mucus, retarded response, feeling of lifelessness, cough and depression[105].

♦ Reasons for *Kapha* Vitiation

Overeating sweet, sour, heavy, oily, moist foods; food containing meat, fish and sesame; sugarcane, milk, salt; eating before digestion of previous meal, sleeping during the day, lack of exercise and physical activity- all these increase *Kapha dosha* in the body. *Kapha dosha* has a tendency to increase naturally during the spring season, in the morning, the first part of the night, after meals and during childhood.

Other foods that increase *Kapha* are curd, milk, sesame, horse bean, milk and rice pudding, sea food, lotus stem, fat, water-chestnut, cocunut, green gourd, pumpkin, and other vegetables that grow on creepers[106].

♦ *Remedies for Aggravated Kapha*:

Taking precaution against the above listed

103. *Ślēşmāa śwētō gurūḥ ṣnigdhaḥ picchhilaḥ śeeta aiva cḥa*
mādhauraṣṭwavidagdhaḥ ṣyāaḍ vidaghō lavaṇaḥ ṣmritaḥ (Su.Su. 21/15)
Gurūśeeta ṃridu ṣnigdha madhura ṣthira picchhilāaḥ
śleṣmaṇaḥ ṗraśamaṃ yāaṇti viprēetaguṇāorguṇāaḥ (Ch. Su.1/61)
śleṣmāahi ṣnigdha ślakṣṇaṃridumadhurasāar sāaṇḍraṃaṇḍaṣtimita
guruśēeta vijjatāaçhhaḥ (Ch. Vi. 8/96)

104. *Śuḳlāakṣaḥ ṣthirakụtitāalinēeklakēśō lakṣmivāaṇ jaladamridaṇgasiṇghaghōśaḥ*
Suptaḥ saṇ sakamalahaṇsa çhaḳravāakāaṇ saṃpaśyēdapi çha jalāaśyāaṇ manōgyāaṇ
Raḳtāaaṇtaneṭraḥ suvibhaḳtagāaṭaḥ snigdhaçhhaviḥ saṭvaguṇōyaṇnaḥ
ḳlēṣakṣmō sāamayitō guruṇāaṃ ggyēyō balāasapraḳritiṛmanuṣyaḥ
Ḍradaśāasṭramitiḥ ṣthiramiṭradhanaḥ pariganya çhirāat pradaḍāatibahu (Sadāa)
Pariniśçhita vāaḳyapadaḥ satataṃ gurumāanakaraṇçha bhavēṭsaḥ sadāa
Brahmarūḍrēṇdravarūṇāiḥ śiṇghāaṣvagajagōvṛiṣāiḥ
Tāarkṣyahaṇsa samāanukaaḥ ślēṣmapraḳratayō narāaḥ (Su.Shā 4/72-76)

105. *Śvāaiṭya śāiṭyakaṇduṣthāṛyagāuravaṣnehasupti ḳledōpdehabaṇdha*
madhuṛyachirakāariṭvāani śtēṣmaṇaḥ kaṛmāaṇi tāiraṇvitaṃ
ślēṣmavikāarameväaḍhyāavaṣyēṭ (Ch. Su.20-18)
Ślēṣmaṇaḥ ṣnehakāathiṇyakaṇdu śeetaṭvagāuravaṃ
baṇdhōpalēpaṣṭāimiṭyaśōphāapaḳṭyatiniḍritāaḥ
Varṇaḥ śwētō rasāu ṣwāadulavanāu çhirkāaritāa (A.H. Su. 12/53/54)

reasons helps keep *Kapha* in balance[107]. The following remedies can be used to restore *Kapha* balance.

1. Using pungent and hot herbal preparations to induce vomiting and as laxatives.
2. Intake of foods that are bitter, pungent, dry, and hot because they have attributes that balance the characteristics of *Kapha dosha*.
3. Intake of foods that have *Kapha*-reducing potency, *Vipak* (taste that emerges after digestion) and effect.
4. Eating honey and pungent alcoholic substances.
5. Medical smoking and fasting (to reduce weight).
6. Different kinds of fomentation (induced sweating) therapy, sun bathing, massage, *ubtan* (smearing herbal paste on body).
7. Exercising- running, sit-ups, swimming etc.
8. Increased sexual activity, staying awake at night, practising martial arts.
9. Wearing warm clothes.
10. *Nāsya* (medication administered through nostrils).
11. Staying active.
12. Keeping up spirits by cultivating positive thinking[108].

Induced vomiting is the best remedy for increased *Kapha*[109] because it clears the vitiated cough from the stomach- the primary *Kapha* site in the body- and the chest area. But it should be ensured the substances used for the process are pungent and hot.

---

106. *Divāaṣwapṇavyāayāanmāala ṣyamadhurāaṃ lalavaṇa śeeta ṣnigdha gurupiçchilābhiśyāaṇdihāayanakaṭhavakanāiṣadhekaṭamāaṣa mahāamāaṣa gōdhōomatilapiṣṭa vikṛiti dadhidugdhakṛiṣrāa Pāayasēkṣuvikāarāanōopāudika māaṃsavasāa visaṃriṇāala Kaśēruka ṣringāataka madhuranallēephala samaśanāaḍhyasana praḅhritibhiḥ ślēṣmāa prakōpamāapaḍyatē* *(Su. Su. 21/23)*

107. *Sakṣēpatah ḳriyāa rāgaḥ nidāanaṃ parivarjaṇaṃ*

108. *Vidhiyukṭāani tēekṣṇōṣṇāanisaṇśōdhanāani rōokṣaprāayāaṇi çhāayāaḅhyavahāaryāaṇi kaṭukatikṭakṣāayōpdhitāani tathāiva dhāavana laṇghana ṗlavana parisaraṇa jāagraṇa niyuḍdha Ṿyavāayavyāayāamōṇmaṛdana snāanōtsāadāanāani viśeṣataṣṭēekṣṇāaṃ Dēerghakāala ṣthitāanāaṃ çha madyāavāayupayōgaḥ sadhōomapāahaḥ suṛvaśaṣvōpavāasaḥ, sukha pratisēdhaścha sukhāarymēvēti* *(Ch. Vi. 6/18)*
Çchiṇnē varōpuṣpaphale ṗrarohāa yathāa vināasaṃ sahasāa ṿrajanti Tathāa hatēsleṣlemaṇi śōdhanēna tajjā vikāarāaḥ praśamaṃ prayāaṇti *(Su. Ch. 33/13)*
madhu çha (sataṭamaḅhyaṣmāanaṃ) ślēṣmāaṇalṃ jayati Rāukṣyāṭtāikṣṇāaṭ kaṣāayaṭvāaçcha ślēmāa hi sṇigdhō maṇdō madhuraṣçha *(Ch. Su. 25/40)*

109. *Vamanaṃ ślāeṣmaharāaṇāaṃ Vamanaṃ tu sarvōpaḳramēḅhyavḥ ślēṣmaṇi pradhāanatamaṃ maṇyaṇtāe bhiṣajaḥ* *(Ch. Su. 20/19)*

♦ Symptoms of Low *Kapha* and Its Treatment

When *Kapha* is low the body displays the symptoms e.g. dryness, a persistent burning sensation, a void feeling in the *Kapha* positions (lungs, heart, joints, and head) looseness of joints, excessive thirst, weakness, lack of sleep. Low *Kapha* affects the normal functioning of the *Kapha dosha*[110].

♦ *Sāam* and *Nirāam Kapha*

When *Kapha* gets corrupted with *āam* (*saam Kapha*), it becomes turbid, dense, sticky and smelly. This obstructs belching and reduces hunger[111]. In contrast, *Nirāam Kapha* is foamy, light, odourless and settled. It does not stick in the throat and keeps the mouth clean and fresh.

♦ Types of *Kapha*

The five types of *Kapha*, on the basis of location and function, are listed below[112]:

Kapha And Its Divisions[113]

S.No.	Type	Location	Function	Illnesses due to vitiation
1.	*Kledak* (moistening)	Stomach	Moistens food and helps in digestion	Poor digestion, feeling of heaviness, common cold, nauseous feeling
2.	*Avalambak* (supporting)	Chest	Energises limbs and heart	Laziness
3.	*Bodhak* (lends perception)	Tongue and throat	Perception of taste	Inability to discern taste
4.	*Tarpak* (satisfying)	Head	Nourishing sense organs	Loss of memory and retardation of sense organs
5.	*Sleshak* (that which connects)	Bone, joints	Lubricating joints to protect, nourish and smoothen movement	Pain in joints and slowing down of their functions

110. *Ślēṣmakṣayē rōokṣatāa aṃtadahi āamāaśayētara ślēṣmāaśayaśōoṇyatāa saṇdhi śāithilyaṃ ṭraśṇāa dāuṛobalyaṃ pṛajāagaraṇaṃ ċha* *(Ch. Su.15/12)*
Taṭra (ślēṣmakśayē) ṣwayōniṛvadhanāaṇyēva pṛatēekāaraḥ Ḅhramōḍvadvēṇṭanāanidrāaṇgamaṛda pariplāeesao tē dadavadāahaśphōtanavēpana dhōomāayana saṇdhi śāithilyaṃ ḥriḍayaḍrava śtēṣmāaśaya śōoṇyatāadibhiḥ ślēṣmāa *(A. Saṇ Su. 21/9)*
111. *Āavilaṣṭaṇṭulaḥ sṭyāanaḥ kaṇthadēśē5atiṣṭhate Sāamo balāasō dwṛgaṇdhaḥ kṣuḍdugāaravidhāata kṛit*
112. *Fēnvāana piṇḍitaḥ pāaṇḍuṛniḥ sāarō5gaṇdha aiva ċha Pakụaḥ sa aivaṃ viggyēyaśḍdēvāaṇ vakṭra śuḍhikṛiti* *(Hri su. 13/27-28 middle)*

6. *Pṛakṛiti* (Constitution)

Each individual is born with a unique body type determined by the dominance of one, or more than one *dosha* in the body. This is the *Pṛakṛiti* or the constitution of the individual. It plays a very important role in determining a person's health, general well-being and treatment to be prescribed at the time of illness. It helps to determine the most beneficial dietary habits and lifestyle that an individual should adopt for a happy and healthy life. Diagnosis of disease and the treatment to be undergone are also dictated by *Pṛakriti*. *Ayuṛvedic* practitioners determine an individual's *constitution* based on his/her body structure, character attributes, nature etc.

The *constitution* of an individual is decided before one is born. A child is conceived in the mother's womb with the fusion of the sperm and the ovum. The *doshas* that are predominant in all three-sperm, ovum and uterus- at the time of conception determine the child's body constitution, its character, nature and mental make- up. These attributes and characteristics are referred to as *Pṛakṛiti* in *ayuṛved*[114]. If all three *doshas* are in balance during conception, the child born is healthy in every respect. On the contrary, if they are completely out of balance, conception will not take place. In case it does, the embryo will either not develop or will be deformed. If one of the three *doshas* dominates, the child's physiological and psychological characteristics will be governed by the dominating *dosha*. If two *doshas* are in dominance, a combination of the qualities of both will determine the *Pṛakṛiti* of the child. There are thus, seven types of *Pṛakṛitis* possible[115]:

1. *Vāta Pṛakṛiti*
2. *Piṭta Pṛakṛiti*
3. *Kapha Pṛakṛiti*
4. *Vāta-Piṭta Pṛakṛiti*
5. *Pitta-Kapha* Prakriti
6. *Vāta-Kapha Pṛakṛiti*

---

113. *Avalaṃbakakḷēdabōdhakataṛpakaśḷēṣakaṭva bhēdāiḥ ṣḷēṣmāa*
Sa tūurathaḥ ṣwavēeryēṇa ṭrikaṣyāaṇna vēeryēṇa ḉha
saha hridayaṣya ḉha śeṣaṇāaṃ ḉha śḷēṣmaṣthāanāaṃ
Taṭraṣtha aivōdakaṛṃaṇāa5valaṃbanāadavalaṃbaka ityuḉhyatē
Amāaśayaṣthitoṇna saṇgāataṣya ḳledanāaṭḳḷēdakaḥ
Rasanāaṣtha seṃyagrasabōdhanāaḍ bōdhakaḥ
Śiraṣthaśḉhkṣurāadēeṇdriyataṛpaṇāaṭ taṛpakaḥ
Paṛvaṣthōssthi saṇdbhiśleṣāaṭ śḷēṣaka iti *(A. H. Su. 20/6)*

114. *Śukraśaṇita saṃyōgce yo bhavēdvōṣa uṭkaṭaḥ*
Pṛakritirjāayatē tēna tasyāa mē lakṣnaṃ ṣruṇu *(Su. Sha, 4/62)*
Kāaladayaṣcha śuḳraśonitamēva kuṛvaṇtaḥ pṛakṛitijanakā
bhavaṇṭēeti taṭrāaṇtarē śuḳtraśoṇitagata dośēṇāiva prakṛiṭyutpāadō daṛśitaḥ *(Chakrapāaṇi)*
Prakṛiti jaṇmapraḅhriti vridhāu ucatāadhih *(Chakrapāaṇi)*

115. *Sapta pṛakritayō bhavaṇti*
Dośāiḥ prithag ḍwiśāiḥ samaṣṭāiṣḉha *(Su. Sha 4/61)*

7. *Sāam Pṛakriti* (Equal effect of all three *doshas*)

It should be noted that although the balance of the *doshas* in an individual shows constant change during the course of his life due to various internal and external factors, the basic *Pṛakriti* is never altered. This means that the dominating *dosha*/s of an individual can be easily aggravated. For example, the slightest disturbance in a *vāta pṛakṛiti* individual increases *Vāyu* immediately. The same is true for all other *pṛakṛitis*[116].

Some of the other factors that affect an individual's *pṛakṛiti* are as follows:

1. Condition of ovum and sperm.
2. Climatic season and condition in the uterus.
3. Food and lifestyle habits of the mother.
4. Attributes of the elements that bring about the fusion of the sperm and ovum.

Pṛakṛiti is also affected by genealogy, ancestry, race (geographical region), time, season, age of the parents especially the mother, and the child's own qualities[117].

Despite being affected by many factors, *Pṛakṛiti* is primarily determined by *doshas*. Hence the *dosha*- based nomenclature. The effects of the three *doshas* on the body have been listed earlier. The characteristics of the three *Pṛakṛitis* (*vāta Pṛakṛiti*, *Piṭta Pṛakṛiti* and *Kaphạ Pṛakṛiti*) are as follows.

---

116. *Aitaāani hiyēna yēna dośēṇ ādhikēnainikāina vāa samanubaḍḍhyaṇtēm*
tēna tēna dośēṇa gaṛbho5nubaḍḍhyatē
tataḥ sāasāa dośakritiruçhyatē manusyāaṇāam garbhāadi pravratāa
Tasmāaçcha śļēṣmatāaḥ prakrityāa kēçhit,
Piṭtaāaḥ kēçhitaa vāatalāaḥ kēçiṭa sanṣriṣṭāa kēçhit (Ch. vi 8/95)

117. *Ṗrokōpē vādaṇyathāabhāavō kṣyō vāa nōpajāayatē*
Pṛakritēenāaṃ swāabhāavēna jāayatē tu gutāmuṣaḥ (Su Sha. 4/77)
Viṣajāatō yathāa kēeṭō na viṣēṇ vipaḍyaṭē
Taḍvaṭ pṛaṛivamō maṛtyaṃ śaknuvaṇti na badhituṃ (Su. Sha. 4/78)

118. *Aḷpakēśaḥ kṛiśō rōokṣō vāachāalaśchalamāanasaḥ*
Āakāaśaçhāaarēe swapanēṣu, vāata pṛakriti ko naraḥ (Sha PU, 6/20)

119. *Akaāalē palitāiṛvyāaptō dhēemana ṣwedēe sha rōṣaṇaḥ*
Ṣwapnēṣujyotiṣêaṃ ḍriṣṭāa, piṭtaprakṛikō naraḥ (Sha PU 6/21)

120. *Gaṃbhēra buḍdhiḥ ṣthōolṇga ṣnigdhakēō mahāabalaḥ*
ṣwapnē jalāṣyāa lōkēe, śļēṣma pṛakriti pṛakriti kō naraḥ (Sha pu 6/22)

121. *Ḍwayōṛvāa tisriṇāaṃ vāapi prakritēenaaṃ tu tēekṣnaih*
jgyaaṭvāa saṇsaṛgajō vāidyaḥ prakritēerabhiniḍviśēṭ (Su Sha 4/76)

122. *Dēhaḍhāaṛaṇāaḍ dhāatavāḥ*
Dhātvō hi dehadhāṛaṇa sāamaṛthyāaṭ saṛvē dośāadaya Uçhchyante (Fram A Sun, Su 1 Indus)
Dhāaqtavō rasa raḳtēmāaṃsa mēdōyanjaśukrāaṇi
tēisāmapi ṣarēerodhārakaṭwāaṭ (Su Chi 5/21 Dalhaṇa)
Raśāasṛingmāaṃsa mēdo5thi majjāa sukrāaṇi dhāatavaḥ sapta dṣyaah (A Ha Su 1/13)

Characteristics of the *Pŗakŗitis*

Vāta Pŗakŗiti[118]	*Piţta Pŗakŗiti*[119]	*Kapha Pŗakŗiti*[120]
Dry and rough Skin Yellowish complexion	Dry and smooth skin. Fair & skin. Fair complexion	Smooth, delicate and soft
Slender, weak frame	Medium build	Physically strong, heavy build.
Short height	Slender and weak muscles	Tendency to be obese
Rough hair, teeth, nails, palms and soles	Loose joints	Strong joints
(Prominent) Veins and tendons hence visible	Profusion of moles and black spots	Prominent forehead, chest and arms
Dry, cracked organs	Very sensitive to heat	
Scanty hair on head and body, beard	Thin and reddish hair	Thick, curly, black hair
Brown hair with split ends	Premature appearance of wrinkles, thinning of hair and balding	
Dry and sleepy eyes	Small & brownish eyes and a few eyelashes	Large beautiful white eyes, Thick eyelashes.
	Enthusiastic and energetic	
	Body odour	
	Blackish tinge on nails, eyes, tongue, Palate, soles, palms and other body part	

People with mixed *Pŗakŗitis*, (like-*vaat, pitta, Kapha*, etc.) display characteristics of both the constituent *doshas*[121].

Vāta Pŗakŗiti people are susceptible to *Vāta* diseases and will easily contract them. The same is true of the other *Pŗakŗitis* as well. Dietary habits and lifestyle that aggravate the dominant *dosha* should be avoided, and habits that keep it in balance should be adopted.

It has been observed that life-span, strength, children, knowledge, material wealth etc. are enjoyed most by *Kapha pŗakŗiti* individuals. *Piţta pŗakŗiti* individuals have these in moderation, while the *Vāta pŗakŗiti* individuals tend to have very little of these.

Knowledge of *Pŗakŗiti* is beneficial to the individual and absolutely essential for a doctor. Medication, diet and lifestyle changes are prescribed keeping in mind the *pŗakŗiti* of the patient because even when the symptoms in two different individuals suffering from the same disease are the same, the medication and diet given to a *piţta pŗakŗiti* individual will be of a cool nature, whereas the medicine and diet prescribed to a *Kapha pŗakŗiti* individual will have hot attributes and taste essence. Only those medicines and foods, which are chosen according to the *pŗakŗiti* of an individual, are beneficial. Others might even aggravate the illness or cause further complications. For example, Quinine is very beneficial for *Kapha pṛaķriti* patients, moderately helpful for *vāta pṛaķriti* patients, but can prove harmful for *Piṭta pṛaķriti* individuals. (The above example proves how essential the knowledge of *pṛaķriti* is to an *ayuṛvedic* practitioner. Hence, a complete knowledge of *pṛaķriti* is an intrinsic part of *ayuṛvedic* system of healing.)

7. Seven *Dhātus*

The most important elements that make up our body are the *dhātus*. They are the basic tissue elements. They form the basic body structure, nourish and sustain it[122]. There are seven types of *dhātus*:

1. *Rasa* or *Lasika* (chyle or plasma)
2. *Raķta (Blood or the haemoglobin part of the blood)*
3. *Māṃsa* (muscle tissue)
4. *Med* or *Vāsa* (fat tissue)
5. *Aṣthi* (bone tissue)
6. *Majjā* (bone marrow)
7. *Shukraa* (Ovum in female and sperm in male)

Like the *doshas*, the seven *dhātus* are also composed of five elements and one or two elements dominate the *Dhātus*[123].

Dhātu	**Dominant element**
Rasa	Water
Raķta	Fire
Māṃsa	Earth
Med	Earth
Aṣthi	Air and Space
Majjā	Fire
Shukraa	Water

The *dhātus* are formed as a result of the action of the *Jathāragni* (digestive fire that breaks down food in the stomach and gastrointestinal tract)[124].

The digestive enzymes break food down into two parts- the *sāar*, (which is nourishing) and the *mala* (which are the waste products and need to be excreted). The *sāar* is carried to different parts of the body by *vyāna vāyu*, where it nourishes and replenishes the *rasa*

123. *Tāaṭra vāayōruāayurēva yōniḥ piṭtaṣyāagni kaphaṣyāapaḥ raķtam tējāajalāaṭmakaṃ, māaṃsa pāaṛthivaṃ mēdāa jalaṗrithivyāaṭmakaṃ, aṣthi ṗrithvyatilāaṭyakaṃ, majjāa śuķraṃ chāaṗyaṃ* *(chakrapami)*

124. *Tatraāśāaṃ saṛvadhāatōonāapāanarasaḥ ṗraṇiyitāa saṗtabhuiṛdedhāatāarō dhāatava dividhapuṇaḥ* *(Su sHA 14/11)*
Yathāaṣwabhagnibhiḥ pāaṇka yāaṇti kiṭta-prasāadavaṭ
Rasāaḍrakạtaṃ tatō māaṃsa maaṃsāaṇmēdaṣtatō5sthi ċha
Aṣthanō majja tataḥ śuķraṃ śukrāadgaṛbhaḥ praśādajaḥ
Rasāḍraķtāṃ tato māaṃsa māaṃsaṇmēdaḥ ṗrajāayatē
Mēdēsāa5ṣthi tato majjāa msjjhaṣḥ śuķra tu jāyāate *(Su. Sri 14/10)*

and *rakṭa dhātus*.

Conversion of food into the building blocks of the body, i.e. the *dhātus*, takes place in a definite order. Food is first converted into *rasa dhātu*, which then makes *rakṭ*, which is then converted to *māṃsa*, *māṃsa* to *med*, *med* into *aṣthi*, *aṣthi* into *majjā*, and finally *majjā* to *shukraa*.

Like *doshas*, the amount of *dhātus* in the body remains constant, and they can be easily corrupted. This corruption or imbalance is a direct result of the imbalance in the *doshas* and leads to illness. The illnesses thus caused are named after the *dhātus* which have been corrupted. Hence, *Rāsaj rog* (ailment of *rasa dhātu*) refers to an illness caused due to corruption of rasa *dhātu*. Similarly there is *Rakṭaj* rog, *Māṇsaj rog*, *Medaj rog*, *Aṣthij rog*, *Majjāgat* rog and *Śhūkrāaj rog*[125]. Given below is a brief description of the natural characteristics and ailments of the seven *dhātus*.

♦ *Rasa Dhātu*

Normal functions: Its main function is to enhance the matter or part where it is located. It produces joy and satisfaction, and helps in manufacturing of the next *dhātu*. i.e. *rakṭ* (blood)[126].

Symptoms of increase: Symptoms similar to *Kapha dosha* vitiation are observed. Other symptoms are decrease in digestive powers, uneasiness, excess salivation, nausea, laziness, heavy feeling, whitening of organs, feeling cold, weakness in limbs, asthma, cough and excessive sleep[127].

Symptoms of Decrease : These include dryness in mouth and other organs, roughness, fatigue, increased thirst, inability to bear loud noises, increased heartbeat, heartache, feeling of emptiness in stomach, heart etc., langour and rapid breathing, and decrease in the amount of other *dhātus*[128].

The causes for increase and decrease of the

---

125. *Dośaadōoṣitēśvaṭyaṛtha dhāatuṣu sanyāa-rasajo5yaṃ śonitōja5yaṃ, māaṃdajē5yaṃ medōjō5yaṃ asthijō5yaṃ majjajō5yaṃ, śkṛajo5yaṃ vyāadhiriti* *(Su sA 24/8)*

126. *Rasaṣtuṣṭi pṛeeṇanaṃ rakṭa puśṭi ḉha karoti,*
Rasē rodayaṃ śramaḥ śoṣāa glāanēḥ śāaṣdāasahiṣṇuṭāa *(Aurndatta)*

127. *rosō5ti vridhāu ḥridayōṭkḷēdaṃ prasēkaṃ chāapāadayati*
ślēmāa (vṛidhāu) sgnisadanaprase kāalaṣyaganu ravaṃ *(Su. Sa 15/19)*
śvāiṭyaśāiṭyaś lathāangaṭwaṃ ṣwāasakāasāatiniḍratāaḥ *(A.h-su. 11/78)*
Rasōs5pi śēṣmavaḍraktaṃ duṛvahāangatwaṃ
śāiṭyaṃ śēetaspaṛśaṃl ṣlathāangaṭwa avayava śāithilyaṃ *(Aurndatta)*

128. *Ghaḍritē sahatē śaḅdaṃ nōḉhachāiṛḍravṛiti śōolayatē*
ḥridayaṃ tāaṃyati ṣwalpaḉhēṣṭasyāapi rasakṣymel *(ch. su. 17/64)*
Rasakṣyēḥṛiṭpēedāakampaśūṇyatāaṣṭriṣṇāa ḉha *(su sa 15/13)*
Rasē (kṣēenē Rāukṣyaṃ ṣramaḥ śośō glāaniḥ śaḅdāasahiṣṇutāa *(A hr. ṣa 11/17)*

rasa dhātu are similar to the causes of aggravation of *Kapha dosha*.

Rasaj rog **:** It causes loss of appetite, general apathy, bad taste in mouth, tastelessness (inability to judge and enjoy taste), pain, fever, fainting, blockage of *srotas* (body channels), impotency, yellowing, thinning, reduction of digestive power, premature wrinkling and graying of hair[129].

♦ *Rakṭ Dhātu (Blood)*

Normal functions: It provides and sustains *Prāṇa* (life breath). It improves colour and makes it possible for sense organs to gather knowledge. *Rakt* nourishes and replenishes *Maṃsa Dhātu*[130].

Symptoms of Increase : Reddening of complexion and eyes, high blood pressure[131]. An increase in the *rakṭ dhātu* can be treated by the therapies of blood-letting and induced nausea[132].

Symptoms of decrease: Weakening of veins, weakening of digestive enzymes, and aggravation of *vāyu*, rough, dull and hard skin, craving for sour and cold foods[133].

The reasons that cause imbalance in *Piṭta dosha* also cause increase and decrease of *Rakṭ Dhātu*.

Rakṭaj rog **:** Leprosy and other skin diseases, erysipelas, pimples, bleeding, bleeding of reproductive organs of females, increased spleen, pseudo tumour, abscess, leucoderma, itching, urticaria, jaundice, gout, and reddening of urine.

The best therapies for the *Rakṭaj rog* are blood-letting and purgation[134].

---

129. *Aśraḍdhāa ċhāruċhiśċhāasya vāraṣyamarasagyatāa*
Hallāasō gāuravaṃ taṇḍrāa sāaṇgamardōjwaraṣtamaḥ
Pāaṇduṭwaṃ ṣrōtaasāaṃ rōdhaḥ kāilyyaṃ sāadaḥ ķriśāuṇgātāa
Nāaśo5śērathāa kāalaṃ balayaḥ paliāaniċha
Rosapradōṣajāa rōgāaḥ (ch. su 27/9-10)

130. *Rakṭaṃ varṇaprasāadaṃ māamsa puśṭe jēevayati ċha*
Teṣaṃ dhāatūnāaṃ) kśyavṛidhēe śoṇitanimiṭtē (Su.sa. 14/21)
Taḍdhi hi rudhairaṃ balavarṇasukhāayuṣāa
Yunakṭi prāaṇinaṃ prāana ṣoṇitaṃ ḥyanuvarṭatē (Ch. Su. 24/4)
Dhāatunaaṃ pōoraṇa varṇaṃ sparśajgāanamasanṣayaṃ
ṣwāah śirāaḥ saṇcharaṛakṭaṃ kuryāaċchhāanyāaṃ guṇāanapi (Su sha 7/14)
Dehaṣya rudhiraṃ mōolaṃ rudhirēnāiva dhāaryatē
Taṣmāghaṭnēna sarakṣyaṃ rakṭaṃ jēeva iti ṣthitiḥ (Su, Sha 14/44)

131. *Rakṭaṃ rakṭāangakṣiṭāaṃ sirāapōorṇaṭwaṃ chċapāadayati*

132. *Kuryāaċhhōṇita rōgēṣu rakṭa piṭtaharēe kriyāaṃ*
Virēkamupavāasaṇchaṣṭrāavaṇaṃ śoṇitaṣya ċha (Ch.Su. 24/18)

133. *Dhaātukḥyāaṭa ṣṭrute rakṭe maṇdaḥ sajāatē5nalaḥ*
Pawanaśċha paraṃ kōpa yati

134. *Kuryāachhōṇitarōgēṣu rakṭa piṭtaharēe kriyāaṃ*
Virēkamupawāasasaṇcha sṭrāvaṇaṃ śōṇitaṣya ċha (Cha Su. 24/18)

♦ *Maṃsa Dhātu*

Functions: *Maṃsa Dhātu*, i.e. the muscle tissue, is the main cementing component of the body. It provides sturdiness and strength to the body. It is involved in the production of *med Dhātu*[135].

Symptoms of increase: Weight gain as a result of accumulation of *muscle* tissue on the neck, hips, cheeks, lips, thighs, legs, calves, stomach, chest etc[136].

In this condition one should adopt therapies that will reduce *Maṃsa* eg. purification, staying awake at night. Foodstuffs made with *ghēe* (clarified butter), oil, animal fats, and sugar must be avoided[137].

Symptoms of decrease: The symptoms due to reduction in *Maṃsa* are opposite to those of an increase. Thinning of the body parts is seen. The patient loses weight and experiences fatigue, roughness, and weakening of blood vessels[138].

To increase muscles, protein rich foods like milk, milk products, sprouted green lentils (*mōoṇg*) and gram (*chana*) should be taken in large quantities. Non-vegetarians will benefit from increased intake of meat and meat broth.

Māṇsaj rog **:** These include accumulation of fat on thighs, goitre, enlarged cervical glands, layer of fat on tongue, palate, neck, etc, tonsils, tumour, warts, development of paunch, swelling of glands, multiple phlyctens (a skin disease), and allergy[139].

Treatment : *Māṇsaj* diseases respond best to surgery, alkalis, cauterization and heat treatment.

♦ *Med Dhātu*

Functions: Providing heat and unctuousness to the body are its main functions. It lends strength and stability to bones. The *Aṣthi dhātu* is made using the *Med dhātu*[140].

---

135. *Māaṃsa śarēerapuṣṭi medasaṣcha (puṣṭiṃ karōti)* *(Su. Sū. 15/7) (i)*

136. *Māaṃsa (ativṛiddhaṃ) ṣphigganḍdāuṣthāupaṣthōrōobāa hujaṇgāanu vṛiddhiṃ gurugāaṭrataaṃ ça (Āapāadayati)* *(Su. Su. 14/15)*

137. *Taṣaṃ yathāaṣuaṃ saṇśōdhanaṃ kṣpaṇaṇça kśyāadvịruchḥaīḥ kriyāaviśeṣsḥ prakurvēeta* *(Su.Su. 15/22)*

138. *Māaṇsakṣyē ṣphiggaṇdośthōpathōrōovakṣaḥ Kṣāapiṇḍikōdaragrēevāa śuṣkatāa rāukṣya todāu gāatrāaṇaam sadanaṃ dḥamanēe śāithilyaṃ ça* *(Su.Su. 15/13)*
Māaṃsakṣyē viśēṣāṇa ṣphiggrēevōdara śuṣkatāa *(Ch. Su. 17/65)*

139. *Adhimāaṃsāarbudāarśō5dhijivḥēpjivḥōpakgalaśuṇdi Kāalēe māaṃsasaghātāuṣthaprakopagalagaṇda gaṇdamāalāa prabhritayō māaṃsadōśajāaḥ* *(Su.sa 25/12*
śoṇita) kśyē ṭwakpāarūśyamaṃla śēeta prāarthanāa sirāa śāithilyaṇchāa *(Su.Sa 15/13)*
Pauṣāa ṣphuṭitāamlāanāa ṭwagrōokśāa raklasaṇkśyē *(Ch. Su. 17/64)*

140. *Mēdah ṣnehaṣwēdāṇ ḍradatwaṃ puṣṭimaṣthāaṃ ça (karoti)* *(Su.Su 15/7)*

Symptoms of increase : Excessive oiliness in the body, symptoms similar to increase in *Maṃsa dhātu* (goiter, development of paunch, etc.), bronchitis, exhaustion, loosening and hanging of buttocks, breasts and stomach due to fat accumulation, increased body odour, etc[141]. All precautions recommended for *Maṃsa* increase should be adopted.

Symptoms of decrease : Pain and feeling of emptiness in the joints, lackluster eyes, skin and hair, blocking of ear etc., fatigue, thinning of body, inability to feel touch on the back, enlargement of spleen etc. The patient craves for fat-rich meal[142].

All therapies for increasing weight are helpful[143].

***Medaj* diseases :** Sweet taste in mouth, burning sensation in limbs and other parts of the body, tangling of hair, laziness, excessive thirst, increased secretion of body wastes like sweat, increased secretion from body pores, numbness in the body[144].

Treatment: An increase in *Med dhātu* can be treated the same way as obesity is cured (fasting etc.). A decrease can be alleviated by following treatment meant to increase weight (increasing intake of fat, oily foods etc.)

♦ *Aṣthi dhātu* (Bone Tissue)

Functions: Constitutes the basic structure (the skeleton) on which the body is constructed and upheld[145] and provides support to the body.

Symptoms of increase: Abnormally large and thick bones, sudden increase in nails and hair mass, and extra teeth[146].

Symptoms of decrease: Pain and loss of sensation in bones and joints, hair fall from body and beard, looseness of joints[147].

***Aṣthijanya* diseases:** Bone enlargement,

---

141. *Mēdaḥ (ativṛidhaṃ) ṣnigḍhaṇgatāamudarapāaṛśwaṿridhiṃ*
Kāasaṣwaāasāadēena dāuṛganḍhyaṇça (Su Su. 15/19)

142. *Sadhēenāaṃ ṣphuṭanaṃ glāanirakṣ̌nōrāayāasa āiva ça*
Lakṣ̌aṇaṃ mēdasi kṣ̌ēeṇē tanuṭwaçhōdaraṣya ça (Ch. Su. 17/66)

143. *Taṭrāapi ṣwayōnā vaṛdhana ḍravyōpayōgaḥ* (Ch. Su. 6/10)
Mēdō mṟedasāa (āapyāayyatē bhōoyaṣtaramaṇyēḅhyaḥ śarēeradhāatuḅhyaḥ) (Ch. Shāa. 6/10)

144. *Granṭhi vṛidhi gala ganḍāaṛbudamēdōjāuṣ́tha pṛakōpa madhu mēhāatiṣthālyāati ṣwēda pṛbhritayō mēdō dōśajāaḥ* (Su. Sū. 24/9)

145. *Aḅhyanṭargatāi sāarāiṛyathāa tiṣ́thanṭi bhōorōohāaḥ aṣthisāarāiṣtathāa dēhāa ḍhriyanṭē dēhināa ḍhruvaṃ* (Su. Shāa. 15/23)
Yaṣmāaçhçhiravinaṣ́ṭēṣu ṭwaṇkmāaṭsēṣu śarēeriṇāaṃ aṣthēeni na vinaśyanṭi sāarāaṇyētaani dēhināaṃ (Su. Shāa 5/21)

146. *Aṣthi (ativṛidhaṃ) aṣthuaḍhyaṣthēeṇyadhidanṭāaṣça (āapāadayati)* (Su. Sū. 15/19)

abnormally large teeth, intense pain in bones and teeth, distortion of nails, diseases of the beard and body hair[148].

Treatment: Increase in bone tissue can be treated through enema with herbal medicines that are bitter. Ailments caused due to decrease in bone tissue respond well to a diet rich in milk, butter milk, cottage cheese, diluted yogurt, dry fruits, pulses, fresh fruits, leafy vegetables, Vitamin D, milk and *ghēe* flavoured with bitter herbs etc. Non-vegetarians can eat medicines prepared from animal bones (for example, tortoise shell ash). Sunlight is also beneficial[149].

♦ *Majjā Dhātu* (Bone Marrow Tissue)

Functions: All bones are packed with bone marrow tissue. Its function is to fill the bones with nourishing fat and provide unctuousness and strength to the body[150].

Symptoms of increase: Heaviness in the body especially the eyes, tenacious boils on the joints[151].

Symptoms of decrease: Hollowness in bones, brittle bones and joints, small and thin physique, dizziness, blackouts, and deficiency of *Shukraa Dhātu* (sperm and ovum)[152].

---

147. *Çhakāarāaṭ kēśanakh5ōrati vṛidhirgyēyāa* *(Dalhan)*
aṭhikṣyē5sthiśōolado daṇtanakhabhaṇgō rakṣyaṃçha *(Su. Sū. 15/13)*
Daṇtabhaṇgō5pi taṭprabhavāaṣthikṣyāadeēva *(chakṛapāaṃ)*
Rāukṣyaṃ dēhaṣya daṇtanakhāanāaṃ çha,
daṇtāardāanāamaṣthimayaṭwāaḍ bhaṇgaḥ *(Dalhan)*
Kēśalōmanakhaśamaṣrū ḍvijaṗrapatanaṃ śramaḥ
jyēyamanakaśyē liṇga sandhiśāithiluyamēva çha *(Ch. Sū. 17/67)*
Bāalaḥ savaṭsarāapannaḥ pāadāḅhyāaṃ yō na gacçhati Sa phaskạ iti uigyēyaḥ *(Kaa ch.)*

148. *Aḍhyaṣthidaṃtāu daṇtāṣthibhēdaśōolaṃ vivaṛnatāa*
kēśalōmanakhaśamaṣṛu dōsāṣçhōṣthipradōṣujāaḥ *(Ch. Sū. 28/16)*

149. *Vaṣtayaḥ kṣēēerasaṛpēeṣitikṭakōpahitāani çha* *(Ch. Su 28/26)*
aṣthikṣyajguāaṇ vaṣtibhiḥ tikṭōpahitāiṣçha kṣēerasaṛpibhiḥ *(A. Saṇgrah)*

150. *Majjāa pṛēeti (pṛēeti) ṣnēha balaṃ śukṛapuṣṭim*
pōoraṇamaṣthānāaṃ çha karōti *(Su. Sū 15/7)*
Mēdō hi saṛvabhōotāanāaṃudaraṣthamaṇvaṣthiṣu çha mahaṭṣu çha majjāa bhavati
Ṣthōoṇāaṣthiṣu viśēṣaṇa majjāa ṭwaḅhyaṇtarēeṣṛataḥ

151. *Majjāa (Suivṛidhiḥ) sevaṇginētragāuravaṃ çha (āapāadyati)* *(Su. Sū. 15/9)*
Tamōdaṛśanamōorçhhāaḅhramapaṛvaṣthōola
mōolāarōorjaṇyanētrāabhiśyaṇda pṛabhritayōyajjadōśajaaḥ *(Su. Sū 24/6)*

152. *Majjakṣya5lpaśukṛatāa paṛvabhēdoṣthini ṣṭōdō5ṣthiśōoṇyatāa çha* *(Su. Sū 15/13)*
Śēeṛyaṇta iva çhāaṣthēehi duṛbalāani laghuni çha
Pṛatataṃ vāatarōgēeni kṣēeṇē majjāani dēhināaṃ *(Ch. Sū 17/68)*

***Majjājaṇya* diseases:** Pain and boils in finger joints, dizziness, fainting and blackouts[153].

Treatment: Intake of all sources of protein bone marrow cures *Majjā* decrease.

♦ *Shukraa Dhātu* (Reproductive Tissues- Sperm and Ovum)

Functions: *Shukraa* is the last *dhātu* and is considered the quintessence sap of all preceding *dhātus*. Its main function is to help in procreation. Patience, courage, fearlessness, sexual attraction, enthusiasm, sturdiness, sexual impulse, easy secretion of seminal fluid etc. are also affected by *Shukraa dhātu*[154].

Symptoms of increase: Secretion of excess semen, increase desire for sex, stones in urethra[155].

Symptoms of decrease: Lack of energy, dry mouth, anaemia, fatigue, impotency, absence of semen secretion during intercourse. Extreme pain in testes and burning sensation in the sexual organs[156].

***Shukraj* diseases:** Impotency, low libido, and cause for unhealthy, impotent, weak and physically/mentally challenged off-springs[157].

Treatment: Increase in *Shukraa dhātu* can be corrected by excess sex and use of and semen decreasing bitter and pungent substances, whereas a decrease benefits from using aphrodisiacs and substances that are sweet.

Increase And Decrease Of *dhātus* : The level of - all seven *dhātus* in the body is controlled by the digestive enzymes known as the *agnis* or the digestive fires[158]. The body has 13 *agnis* in all, out of which seven are

---

153. *Rōokra paṛvaṇāaṃ ḅhramō mōorçhhāadaṛśanaṃ tamasatathāa*
arūṣāaṃ ṣthōolamōolāanaaṃ paṛvajāanāaṃ ça daṛśanaṃ
mayjāa ṗradōṣāaṭ (Ch. Sū 17/68)

154. *Śuķraṃ ḍhāiṛyaṃ çhyavanaṃ ṗrēetimḍēhabalaṃ haṛṣa*
(Karoti) bēejāaṛthançha (Su. Sū 15/7)
Dhāiṛya Śāuṛyaṃ śōoraṭwaṃ, ataivaṃ ķlēenāa adhēerāah
dēhabalamuṭsāahāpaçhaya lakṣanaṃ (Dalhan)

155. *Śuķraṃ (ativṛidhaṃ) śuķrāaśmarēe5tiṗrāaduṛbhāavaṃ ça (āapāadayati)* (Su. Sū 15/8)

156. *Dāuṛbaḷya mukhaśōṣaṣça paanḍuṭwaṃ sadaṃ śramaḥ*
Ķlāiśyaṃ śuķrāavisaṛgaṣça ķṣēeṇa lakṣaṇaṃ (Ch. Sū 17/69)
Śuķrakṣyē mēḍravṛiṣaṇa vēdanāa5śakṭi māithunē çhirāaḍvāa
Ṗrasēkaḥ, ṗraśēkē çhāalparakṭaśuķra ḍarśanaṃ (Su. Sū 15/13, Su. Shā 4/12/13)

157. *Śuķraṣya dōṣāaṭ ķlāivyamahaṛṣaṇaṃ*
Rāagi vāa ķlēebamalpāayuṛvirōopaṃ vāa prajāayatē (Ch, Sū 28/18)
Na çhāasya jāayatē gaṛbhaḥ patati ṗraṣravaṭyapi
Śuķra hi duśṭaṃ sāapaṭyaṃ Sāadarabāadhātē naraṃ (Ch. Sū 28/119)
Ķlāivyāa ṗrahaṛṣa śukāaśmarēe śuķra dōṣāadayaṣça taḍḍōṣajāah (Su. Sū. 24/7)

158. *Bhāutikāaḥ pançha, dhāaṭwagnayaḥ sapta, aṇnapakṭāa āikaḥ*
kivāa, āṗraḍhāaṇyadaṇyāaṇyakiviṇṭkrāaṇi nōķṭāani (Chaķrapāaṇi)

dhātu-agnis, or *Dhātvāgṇis*. If the *Dhātvāgṇis* are in balance, the *dhātus* will remain in balance[159]. When the *Dhātvāgṇis* become too active, then there starts a decrease in the *dhātus* due to excessive metabolism of food which is the primary source for the regenaration of all seven *dhātus*. In contrast, weak *Dhātvāgṇis*, will lead to an increase in the *dhātus* and poor digestion . With a change in the level of each *dhātu*, all other *dhātus* are changed as one is formed from the other in a chain-like process[160]. Therefore, to keep the *dhātus* in balance, it becomes imperative to keep the seven *Dhātvāgṇis* in balance.

8. *Ojas*

In the transformation of food from *rasa* to *shukra dhātu*, every step releases *ojas*[161]. It is the essence of all the *dhātus* and it is also referred as *bala*. Just as bees collect honey from flowers[162], the digestive fires collect *ojas* from the *dhātus*. Like *dhātus, ojas* is also nourished by *āhār ras* (the nourishment-rich product of the metabolic process on food). Even though it permeates the entire body, it is located in the heart[163], from where the arteries carry and distribute it throughout the body.

Ojas is moist and unctuous and has a reddish, yellowish and whitish hue. It is of two types[164]:

1. *Par* : Located in the heart, its normal amount is eight points. Its absence leads to death[165].

2. *Apar* : Spread over the entire body, its normal amount is about a handful. A decrease in the *apar oja* leads to lifelessness, indifference and reduced immunity.

---

159. *Ṣwaṣthāanaṣya kāayāagnērasāaṃ ḍhāatuṣu saṇṣritāa*
Teṣāaṃ sāadāatidēeptibḥyāaṃ dhāatu ṿridhikṣyōḍravaḥ (A. h. Su. 11/34)

160. *Samadōṣāaḥ sāamāagniśçha samadhāatuḥ malakṛiyāa*
Ṗrasaṇṇāaṭmēṇḍriyamanāaḥ ṣwaṣtha itiyabhēedhēeyatē (Su. Sū 15)

161. *Rasāadēenāaṃ śukṛāaṇṭāanāaṃ dhāatunāaṃ yaṭparaṃ tējaṣtaṭ*
Kalyōjaṣvadēva balamiṭyuçhyatē, ṣwaśāaṣtra siḍḍhāantāaṭ (Su. Sū 15/23)
Tadāiva saṛvāaṇ dhāatunanupraviṣṭaṃ tēṣāaṃ prabhāavaviśaya
-māadadhāanaṃ taṭṭeja uçhyatē (A.h. Su. 11/37)

162. *Taṭparaṣyāujasaḥṣthāanaṃ taṭra çhāitaṇyasaṇgrāḥaḥ*
ḥridayaṃ māhadarthaśçha taṣmāaduḳtaṃ çhikiṭsakāiḥ (Ch. Sū 30/7)
Tēna bhōolēna mahatāa mahāamōolāa malāa dōśa
ōjōvahāaḥ śarēere5ṣmiṇ vidhaṃyaṇtē samaṇtataḥ

163. *Ḅhraṃrāaḥ phalapuśpēḅhyō yathāa saḅhriyatē madhu*
Tadvaḍḍōjaḥ śarēerebhyō guṇāiḥ saḅhriyatē ṇriṇāaṃ (Ch. Sū 17/16)

164. *Rasavāatāadimāaṛgāaṇaaṃ saṭwabuḍviṇḍriyāaṭmanāaṃ*
Ṗradhāanaṣyāujasaṣçḥāiva ḥridayaṃ ṣthāanamuçhyatē (Ch. Chi 24/35)

165. *Ṗrāṇāaṣṛayaṣyāujasāu5ṣṭāu biṇdavō ḥridayāaṣritaaḥ iti*
Aṛḍhāajjalēe parimitaṣyāanjaṣo ḍhmaṇya aivaṃ ḥridayāaṣrit ṣthāanamḥ

♦ **Functions of *Oja* and its importance**: *Oja* lends strength and radiance to the body. Being the essence of all *dhātus*, its decline in the body, leads to a corresponding decline in the ability of the *dhātus* to support the body, even when they are in balance[166]. It keeps all *dhatus* steady and nourished. All physical, mental, sensory and motor functions are made possible by *ojas*. In times of joy and sorrow it is also the source of will power, determination, patience and enthusiasm. It refines speech and complexion, and strengthens immunity. It is the foundation of a health and happiness .

Some experts consider *ojas* an upa *dhātu* (minor *dhātu*), but being found in infinitesimal quantities, it is unable to nourish and sustain any one single *Dhātu*[167].

♦ **Symptoms of decrease :** A timid and scared personality, dry and lustre-less appearance, a general listlessness, weakness in the mind and body, worries and tensions, painful and fatigued organs, and a loss of zest for life[168].

♦ **Causes of decrease :** Anger, worrying, fear, sorrow and other psychological excitements; decline in the amounts of *dhātus*, *doshas*, or *malas*; excessive fasting or inadequate diet; eating and drinking too many rough, dry and harsh foods; overwork; insomnia; excessive secretion of *Kapha*, *mala*, blood and semen; emaciation due to sickness; and external injury – all can lead to a decline in *ojas*[169].

♦ **Treatment:** Use of sweet, cold, moist, oily, light and wholesome foods; milk, meat soup, life-prolonging herbal preparations, *aṣhwagaṇdha*, and other rejuvanatiing medicines; aphrodisiacs helps to increase the amount of *ojas* in the body. In addition, keeping oneself happy and adopting health promoting diet and lifestyle also boosts *ojas*[170]. Keeping *srotas* (channels) of *malas* and *dhātus* clean is also important. An increase in the *ojas* results in contentment, joy, physical & mental strength. A surplus of *ojas* is beneficial and does not lead to any illness.

Children should be encouraged to adopt diet and lifestyle that boost *ojas*.

166. *Tatra balēna ṣthirōpaçhitamāa ṃsātāa saṛvaçhēṣṭāaswapratiġhāatah*
Swaṛvaṛna pṛasāadō bāahyāanāabhāaḅhyanṭarāaṇāam
kāaṛaṇāanāaṃāaṭmakāaṛya pṛatipaṭṭiṛbhavati *(Su. Sū 15/25)*

167. *Āitaçhçhāuçha upadhāaturōopa kēçhidāaḥaḥ, dhāaturḥi*
dhāaraṇapōṣaṇayōġāaḍ bhavati, ōjaṣtudehadhāarakaṃ sadapi
na dēha pōṣakaṃ tena nāaṣṭamō dhāaturōjaḥ *(Ch. Su. 30/7 Chkrapāaṇi)*

168. *Ōjōkṣya ke lakṣaṇa*
Ōjaḥ saṇkṣēeyatē kōpakṣuḍvaḥ yāanaśoka ṣramāadibhiḥ
Vibhēti duṛbalōḍbhēekṣṇaṃ ḍhyāayati ṿyathitēṇḍriya *(AS. 38)*

169. *Abhighāatāaṭ kṣyāaṭ kōpāaçhhō kāaḍ ḍhyāanāaçhhramāaṭ kṣuḍhaḥ*
Ōjaḥ saṇkṣēeyatē ḥyēṃyōdhāatu grahaṇāani ṣritaṃ *(Su. Sū 15/28)*
Dhāatavō grahaṇṭē yāiṣṭāani dhāatugrahaṇāani ṣṭrotāasi ōjōvāahini
Kivāaṃ dhāatugrahaṇaṣtrōtaḥ ṣthāanatayāa dhāatugrahaṇaṃ ḥridayaṃ *(Chakṛapāaṇi)*

9. *Upa-Dhātus*

Those components of the body that lend support and structure, but being present in small quantities, do not participate in the production of other *dhātus*, are called *upa-dhātus*. The major difference between *dhātus* and *upa-dhātus* is that *dhātus* not only support the body but also regenerate the next *dhātu*, where as *upa-dhātus* only share the task of lending support to the body They are named *upa-dhātus* because they are produced from *dhātus*[171]

Nourishment of *Upa-dhātus*

Just as the *ras dhātu* produces the *rakṭ* (blood) *dhātu*, it also produces milk and menstrual blood. While blood is produced regularly, menstrual blood is produced only once in a month[172].

In the same way, *rakṭ dhātu* not only produces *māṃsa dhātu*, it also nourishes the veins and the arteries. Similarly, *māṃsa* and *med dhātu* produce not only *med* and *aṣthi* respectively, but also nourish nerves, ligaments and joints. Breast milk, menstrual fluid, arteries, veins, fat, skin, nerves are the seven *upa-dhātus*.

A brief description of three main *upa-dhātus* is given below:

1. Skin[173]

Skin covers the entire body. It helps body perceive sensations such as heat, cold, light, heavy, hard, soft etc.

---

170. *Jēevanēeyāuṣadha kṣēerarasāadhāaṣtaṭra bheṣajaṃ* (A.H. Su 11/41)
Madhuraṣnigdhaśēetāaṇni laghuni ċha hitāani ċha
Ōjasō varḍhanāaṇyāahuṣtaṣmāadvāa bāalāaṣthatāa55śayēṭ (Ka. Sū 27/16)
Taṇmahaṭ tāa mahāamōolāaṣta ċhchāujaḥ parikṣatāa
Parihaṛyāa viśēṣēṇa manasō dukhahēṭavaḥ (Ch. Sū 30/13)
Ōjaṣtu tējō dhāatunāaṃ śukraṇtāanāaṃ paraṃ ṣṃritaṃ
ḥridayaṣthamapi Vyāapi dēhaṣthitinibaṇdhanaṃ (A.h. Su. 11/37)
Dēhaḥ sāavayanaṣtēna Vyāaptō bhavati dehiṛnāaṃ
Taḍabhāavāaċcha śēeṛyaṇtē śarēerāaṇi śarēeriṇāaṃ (Su. Sū 15/26)

171. *Tē ċha ṣtāaṇyāadayō dhāaṭvaṇrāapōṣaṇāahrēepapōṣakāḥ*
api upadhāatu śaḅdēnōċhyaṇtē
Rasāadayaṣtu śarēeradh1aarakatāayāa dhāaṭvaṇtarapōṣakatayāa
ċha dhāatu śaḅdēnōċhyaṇtē (Chakrapaaṇi)

172. *Rasāaṭ ṣtaṇya tātō raḳtamaṣrija kaṇḍarāaḥ śirāaḥ*
Māaṃsāaḍvēsāa ṭwaċhaḥ ṣaṭa ċha mēdasaḥ ṣnāayuṣaṃbhavaḥ (Ch. Chi 15/17)
Rasāadēv ṣtriyāaṃ raḳtaṃ rajaḥ sangyaṃ pravaṛtatē (Su. Sū 14/7)
Sirāa ṣnāayurajaḥ ṣtaṇya ṭwachō gatiṛvivaṛjitaaḥ
Dhāatuḅhyaśċhōpajāayaṇtē taṣmāaṭ upadhāatavaḥ iti (Chakrapaani)

173. *Etāaḥ (ṭwaċhaḥ) Ṣadangaṃ śiarēemavataṭya tiṣ́thaṇt*
Lakṣnaṃ saṛvamēvāitaṭ ṣpaṛśanēṇhiyagōċharaṃ (Ch. Sha 7/4)

♦ **Physical structure**

Even though it has all the five elements, the element of air predominates. This is why it takes on the tactile quality of air.

♦ **Function:** Apart from tactile functions, the skin keeps the *vāyu* of the body normal; it helps absorb nutrients applied on skin and lends lustre. Sweat glands are also embedded in the skin.

2. Breast Milk

This is found only in females. Breast milk is the best nutrition for new born babies. Hence, it is termed life-giving[174]. It is produced from the sweet parts of the *āhār ras*, and like *shukra* it is present in the entire body. It reaches the breasts when required. Healthy and nourishing, breast milk mixes easily with water, is sweet, yellowish and odourless. A decrease in this *upa-dhātu* can be corrected with increased intake of *kapha* liquids. Cumin seeds, *shatavari* etc. also help improve milk formation. Abundance of breast milk should be treated by purification (draining by suckling or breastpump) and taking light liquids[175].

3. Menstrual Fluid[176]

This is also a female-specific *upa-dhātu*. After attaining is age of 12 puberty, menstrual fluid is discharged from the female body once a month. . Normally it lasts for three to five days. Between the ages of 40 and 50 this discharge ceases. This is called menopause.

Its main function is to prepare the womb for pregnancy. Its characteristics are similar to that of blood[177]. Fluid discharged once a month without pain or burning feeling, is neither too much or too little, has the colour of a red lotus, which easily washes off clothes, and lasts for not more than five days, is considered healthy[178].

Excessive bleeding, body ache and odourous fluid results from an increase in the *upadhātu*. It leads to loss of weight and swelling of the abdomen. During a decrease, the bleeding is delayed and reduced, and leading to pain in the genital organs[179].

---

174. *Ṣtaṇyaṃ ṣtanayōrāapēenaṭwajananaṃ jēevanaṃ ċheti* *(Su. Sū 15/9)*
Jēevanaṃ balāanāam, teṣamēva ṣtrēekṣēerasāatmayaṭwāat *(Dalhau)*

175. *Yaṭ kṣēeramudakē kṣēepṭamēki bhavati pāaṇḍuraṃ*
madhuraṃ chāavivaṛna ċha ṗrasaṇna taḍviniṛdiśēṭ *(Su. Ni. 10/26)*
Ṣtaṇyasaṃpaṭ ṭu ṗrakritvaṛṇagandharasaspaṛśaṃ
Udamapāatrē duhanamāanamudakaṃ vyēti ṗrakṛiti
bhōotaṭwāaṭ taṭ puṣṭikaramāarōgyaṃ ċheti

176. *Rasāadēv rajaḥ ṣtrēeṇaaṃ māasi māasi gyaṇha ṣstravēṭ*
taḍ vaṛṣāaḍ ḍvadaśāadōoṛḍhva yāati paṇchāaśatah kṣyaṃ *(Su. Sa)*

177. *Raktalakṣaṇmāaṛtava garbhakṛiċhcha*

178. *Māasāanniśpiċhhadāahāaṛti paṇcharāaṭranubaṇḍhi ċha*
Nāivāati bahu nāatyalpamāaṛtavaṃ śuḍhamāadiśēṭ *(Ch. Chi. 30/225)*

179. *Āaṛtavaṃ (ālivaṇḍṿa) angamaṛdamati ṗravṛiti dāurgaṇḍhyaṃ ċha* *(āapāadayati)*
Aaṛthva ṿridhatayāa vāatarōdhāaḍaṇgmarda karōti *(Chakrapāani)*

10. *Mala Padāṛth* (Body Wastes)

The metabolic action on food results into two products- *sāar* from which *dhātus* are nourished and regenerated, and *asāar* from which body wastes such as stool, urine, sweat etc. are produced. These waste products are called *malas* (from *malēen* which means befouling) [180]. Since they are contaminated (dóshit) by *vāyu*, they are also termed *dūṣhya*. Regular expulsion of these *malas* is of utmost importance for good health.

Apart from the undigested part of the ingested food, the *malas* also contain toxins produced by tissue sacs (*ūtak koshan*) during metabolic activity, during digestion, dead and lifeless tissues, vitiated *Vāta*, *Piṭta*, and *Kapha doshas*, and other toxins produced by the body.

On accumulation, the *malas* move towards the rectum, bladder, sweat glands and other excretory organs for expulsion from the body. Stool, urine, sweat, nails, hair, facial hair (moustache and beard), body hair, and the secretions from nose, ear, eyes, mouth (like cough, ear wax etc.) are all waste products. A brief description of the three main *malas*- stool, urine and sweat- is given below[181].

♦ Stool (*Purēeśh*)

Stool constitutes the undigested part of ingested food (*asāar*) and the waste produced by the tissue cells. This is why a person who hasn't eaten for many days, and even the baby in the womb also produce stool. It is hence imperative that the stool be regularly expelled from the body in order to enable the tissue cells to remain healthy. When stool is not regularly and properly removed from the body, diseases like backache, rheumatism, sciatica, paralysis, bronchitis and asthma are easily contracted. Therefore the first medicine for all these ailments is a laxative to clean out the bowels. Apart from these, accumulation of *mala* in the bowels encourages growth of worms and other harmful microbes. These often prevent other useful microbes from benefiting the body. Therefore, it is essential that the body be cleansed regularly and all waste products expelled on time[182].

♦ Functions Of Stool

Removal of *Purēeśh* or stool provides support and tone to the body, and bears *Vāyu*

---

180. *Malinēe karaṇāadāahāaramalaḷyāaṇmalāa* *(A.h. Su 1/13)*

181. *Kiṭṭamaṇnaṣya viṇmōoṭraṃ tu kaphō5ṣrijaḥ*
Piṭta māaṃsaṣya khamalāa malaḥ ṣwēdaṣtu mēdasaḥ *(Ch. Chi 15/18)*
Kaphaḥ piṭtaṃ malaḥ khēṣu ṣwēdaḥ ṣyāaṇnakharōma ḉha
Neṭraviṭ ṭwaķśu ḉha ṣnēhō dhāatōonāaṃ ķramaśō malāaḥ *(Su. Sū 46/57)*

182. *Purēeṣamupaṣtaṃbhaṃ vāayvagnidhāaraṇaṃ ḉha* *(Su. Sū 15/8)*
Purēeṣaķśyē ḥridaya pāaśva pēedāa saśaḅdaṣya ḉha
Vāayōrōoṛvagamanaṃ kukśāu saṇḉharaṇaṃ ḉha *(Su. Sū 15/15)*
Ķśēeṇē śaķriti ḉhāaṇtrāaṇi pēedayaṇniva māarutaḥ
Rōokśaṣyōṇnamayaṇ kuķśiṃ tiṛyagōoṛḍhva ḉha gaḉhhati *(Ch. Su 17/70)*

and *Agni*. Patients of tuberculosis, who suffer from a decrease in all *dhātus*, are supported by energy from stool and it is ensured that such patients do not pass excess stool. The slightest increase in stool elimination results in severe weight-loss in such patients.

Excess stool causes shooting pains, bloating, unsettled bowels, and a feeling of heaviness. Overeating causes indigestion[184].

When there is deficient production of stool, *Vāyu* causes spasms in the intestines and moves upwards. The deficiency occurs due to diarrhoea, passing of excessive stool and eating less than required.

To increase stool, foods like horse bean, *Green gram*, barley, leafy vegetables, flour with husk, and fibrous foods must be eaten in larger quantities[185].

♦ Urine

Urine also aids in expulsion of wastes from the body. It is the liquid part of *asāar* (undigested part of food). Its helps expel excess water[186]. Plenty of water should be drunk both in summers and winters to maintain good health. This will help in passing urine atleast 6 times a day and also expel toxins from the body.

Passing too much urine is also a kind of disease. This causes pain and bloating, a feeling of heaviness, restlessness and discomfort due to frequent urination. These symptoms also occur when the urge to pass urine is suppressed, or water is taken during the urge[187].

Decrease in urine production causes a pricking pain in the urethra, When very little urine is eliminated, pain is felt during urination, its colour becomes yellowness or sometimes blood appears with urine, excessive thirst and dry mouth[188] is experienced. Sugarcane-juice, liquids, foods that are sweet, sour and salty increase the quantity of urine[189].

---

183. Śuķorayaţtaṃ balaṃ puņsāaṃ malāayaţtaņçha jēevanaṃ
Toşmāadyaţnēna saņrakşyē yakşmiņō malarťasēe *(Yo. Ra. bhāi. Ra)*
Purēeşamupaşţambhaṃ vāayvagniḍhāaraṇaṃ çha *(Su. Sū 15/8)*

184. Purēeşamāatōpaṃ kukśāu śōolaṃ çha *(Su. Sū 15/20)*
Kukśāavāadhmāanamāatōpaṃ gāuravaṃ vēdanaṃ śakrita *(A.h. Su. 11/13)*

185. Taţrāapi şwayōnivaŗdhana ḍravyōpayōgaḥ pratikāaraḥ *(Su. Sū. 15/14)*
Purēeşakśyē kulṃāaşamāaşamāaşakuşkuņḍāajamaḍhyayaśāaka
-dhāaņyāaṃlāanāaṃ *(Ch. Shāa 6/11)*

186. Āahāraşya rasaḥ sāaraḥ sāarahēenō malaḍravaḥ
Śirāabhişţajjalaṃ nēetaṃ vaşţāu mōotraţwamāapnuyāaţ *(Shāa. Pū 6/6)*
Paķvāamāaśayamaḍhyaşthaṃ piţtaṃ çhatuŗvidhamaņna
- pāanaṃ paçhati, vivēçhayati çha dośarasamōoţrapurēeşāaṃ *(Su. Sū - 21/10)*

187. Mōoţraṃ mōoţravridhiṃ muhuŗmuhuḥ pravŗitiṃ
Vaşţitōdayamāaḍhmāanaṃ çha *(Su. Sū. 15/20)*

188. Mōoţrakşyē vaşţitōdō5lpamōoţratāa çha *(Su. Sū 15/15)*
Mōoţrakśyē mōoţrakŗiçhhraṃ mōoţravīvaŗyamēva çha
Pipāasāa bāadhatē çhāaşya mukhaṃ çha parisuśyati *(Ch. Sū 17/71)*

♦ Sweat

Sweat is a very important *mala*[190]. Sweating is essential for keeping the skin healthy and expelling waste products. It aids the skin in regulating body temperature during different seasons.

Heat, exercise and physical work lead to sweating. On coming in contact with air the sweat evaporates, lowering the body temperature. In contrast, during winters, the body does not sweat and maintains the temperature.

Although the body sweats round the year, it is felt only when it is in excessive quantity or under humid conditions. Excessive sweat causes the skin to smell and itch[191]. Less sweat causes blockage of pores, drying and cracking of skin, loss of tactile perception and body hair[192]. Massage, exercising, staying away from windy places, induced sweating (*svedana*), consuming foods that cause sweating (honey-water etc.) taking sweat-producing and hot medicinal preparations – are helpful in increasing sweat[193].

It is clear that even though they are waste products, *malas* are essential for the upkeep of a healthy body.

♦ Other Waste Products

The above statement is true of the other wastes produced in the eyes, ears, mouth, nose and other body parts. These should be produced just enough to maintain the required moisture in these organs. On increased production, these body parts feel heavy and there is increased secretion. A decrease in the levels of these *malas*, dryness, pain, lightness and emptiness is experienced. Increase is caused due to accumulation, and a decrease due to too much secretion.

Even though both an increase as well as a decrease are harmful, the latter is more detrimental because in this condition they are unable to support and help the organs perform their normal functions.

---

189. *Aṭrāapi ṣwayōnivaṛdhanaḍravyāaṇi pṛātēekāarah̩* *(Su. Sū 15/15)*
Mōoṭrakṣ́yē punnarikṣ́urasavāarōoṇēe maṇḍaḍravamadhurāaṃ
- lalavaṇōpakḷēdināaṃ *(Ch.Shā 6/11)*

190. *Malaḥ ṣwēdaṣtu mēdasāḥ* *(Ch. Chi 15/18)*
Ṣwēda vahāanāaṃ ṣrōtasāam mēdō mōolaṃ lōmakōopāaṣ́ḉha *(Ch. 5/8)*

191. *Ṣwēdaṣṭwaḉhō dāuṛgaṇḍhyaṃ kaṇdōoṃ ḉha* *(Su. Sū 15/20)*

192. *Ṣwēdakṣ́yē ṣtaḅḍha rōmakōopatāa ṭwakṣ́oṣaḥ*
Ṣwaṛśavāiguṇyaṃ ṣwēdanāa saṣ́ḉha
āḅhyaṇgaḥ ṣwēdōpyōgaṣ́ḉha *(Su. Sū 15/15)*
Ṣpaṛśavāiguṇyamiti ṣwēdakṣ́yē vriḍḍrivāatēna jgyēyaṃ
Ṣtaḅdharōmakōopatāa ṣwēdakṣ́yēṇa teṣāaṃ śuśkaṭwāaṭ
Swēdē rōmaḉhyutiḥ, ṣtaḅḍharōmatāa, sphuṭanaṃ ṭwaḉhaḥ *(A.Sam. Sū 11/12)*

193. *Ṿyāayāamāadatisaṇṭāapāaḉhhēetōṣṇāakṛamasēvanāaṭ*
Ṣwēdavāahēeni duśyaṇti ḳrodhaśōkabhayāiṣṭathāa *(Ch. Vi. 5/22)*

The *malas* are naturally odorous, but unbearable smell is an indication that something is out of balance and needs attention.

♦ *Doshas*, *Dhātus* And *Malas*

These three together form the foundation of the human body being the building blocks and primary sustainers[194]. Hence their relation with each other and interdependence is of prime importance. The relationship between *doshas* and *dhātus* is that of supporter and dependent. For example, *Vāyu* is located in *Aṣthi dhātu (bone)*, *Piṭta* in *Rakṭ (blood)* and *Svedā dhātus*, and *Kapha* in the remaining *dhātus*. The treatments prescribed for the balancing of *doshas* has a direct impact on the *dhātus* they reside in. The only exception to this is the *Vāyu dosha* and the *Aṣthi dhātus* where it resides. Normally, an increase in the *doshas* and *dhātus* is treated with fasting and satiating *(tarpan)* therapies, and a decrease with nourishing or filling/ gratifying/satiating therapies. The therapies recommended for *Vāyu* imbalance are opposite.

11. Digestion and Metabolism

The proteins, carbohydrates, oils, vitamins, etc. are ingested as food, nourish the *dhātus*, and provide strength, colour, intelligence, longevity etc. But this is possible only when the ingested external elements are successfully converted into body elements. This entire process is called digestion and metabolism, and the substances that carry-out these processes are referred to as *agnis*[195]. Different enzymes are produced by these *agnis* in the stomach, liver and *dhātu* channels to carry out digestion. These enzymes convert all solid, semi-solid and liquid foods to *dhātus* and *malas*. Although *Vyāna Vāyu*, which carries digested food material all over the body, and *Srotas* (channels) that transport and distribute nourishment, are very important for the digestive process, the *jathār-agni* is the most significant. Without it, neither can food be digested nor *dhātus* produced. If the *agni* is

---

194. *Dōśa dhāatu malamōolaṃ hi śarēeraṃ* (Su. Sū 15/3)
Dośa dhāatu malāa mōolaṃ sadāa dēhaṣya (A.hr. Su 11/1)
Ṿrikṣ̌aṣya ṣkaṇdhaśāakhāadiyukṭaṣṭaṣya mōolaṃ p̣radhāanaṃ
Tadāarabḍhāaṭ, tathāa dēehaṣya dośa dhāatumalāaḥ (Arundatta)
Ṭrayō dośāa dhāatavaśc̣ha purēeṣaṃ mōoṭramēva c̣ha
dēhaṃ saṇdhāarayaṇṭyētē ḥyavỵāapaṇnāa rasāiṛhitāiḥ (Su. U. 66/67)
Dosaadēeṇ vaṛjayiṭwāa nāaṇyac̣hharēera saṃbaḍḍhaṃ śarēerē daṣ̌yate
Ta aivaṃ saṇyukṭāadēha iti yāavaṭ (A.Sa.Sū. 16 in indu)

195. *Balamāarōgyamāayuṣc̣ha p̣rāaṇāaṣchāagnāu p̣ratiṣ̌thitāaḥ* (Ch. Su. 27/342)
Agṇāu p̣ratiṣ̌thitāa iti agṇyaṛdhāaḥ ap̣rāaṇāariti vāayavaḥa
Yadaṇnaṃ dēhadhāaṭvōjōbalavaṛnāadipōṣakaṃ
Taṭrāagniṛhēturāahāarāaṇna ḥyapakẉāaḍ rasāadayaḥ (Ch. Chi 15/5)

destroyed, it becomes fatal. If it gets corrupted, it leads to ailments. When it is normal and balanced, it supports a long and healthy life[196].

Types of *Agnis*

There are in all 13 types of *agnis*:

1. *Jathārāgni*
2-8. *Dhātvāgnis*
9-13. *Paṇch Bhutāgnis*[197]

♦ *Jathāragni*

The *agni* spoken of above is the *Jathāragni*. It is also called digestive-fire *(Pāçhakagni)* or *Kāyāgni*. It is located in the stomach and the navel area between the large and the small intestines[198]. Just as the Sun uses its rays to evaporate water from ponds, lakes and rivers, the *Jathāragni*, from its location in the navel, digests food as soon as it is consumed. All that we eat is broken down into smaller units and transformed into substances that are analogous to body constituents.

Hence, the main functions of the *Jathāragni* is to initiate the metabolic process and support age, complexion, voice, strength, energy, physical growth, enthusiasm, *ojas*, body temperature and the other *agnis* and keep them functional[199]. To be able to carry out these functions it needs to be in balance. *Jathāragni* can be classified in the following four states :

a. *Vishmāgni*

As its name suggests, this type of *Jathāragni* is never stable. It oscillates between high and low intensity and is occasionally in balance. Digestion is thus fast, slow or normal according to its state. This state of *Jathāragni* occurs due to an increase in the *Vāyu dosha*. It results in stomach ache, constipation, heaviness in the stomach,

---

196. *Rōgāaḥ saṛvēśpi maṇḍē5gnāu* *(A.hr. Ni. 12/1)*
Samaprakōpāu dōśāaṇaaṃ saṛvēṣāamagnisaṇṣ́ritāu
Taṣmāadagniṃ sadāa rakṣ́ēṇnidāanāani ça varjayēṭ *(Ch. Chi 5/136)*

197. *Bhāumāapyāagnēyavāayavyāaḥ paṇchōṣmāaṇaḥ sanāabhasāaḥ*
Paṇchāahāarguṇāaṇ ṣwāaṇ ṣwāaṇ pāaṛthivāadēeṇ paçhaṇti hi *(Ch. Chi 15/13)*
Yathāaṣvēnōṣmaṇāa pakaaṃ śarēerāa yāaṇti dhāatavaḥ
Ṣtrōtasāa ça yathāaṣwēna dhāatuḥ puṇyati dhāatuṭaḥ *(Charak)*

198. *Taṭra, paķwāamāaśayamaḍhyagaṃ tatraṣthmēva piṭṭāanāa*
śēṣāaṇāamapyanugrahaṃ
Karoti baladāanēna 'pāachakaṃ' nāam taṭṣṃritaṃ *(A. hr. Su 12/10-12)*
Yaṣtaṃ çhikiṭsēṭ sēedaṇtaṃ sāiva kāayaçhikiṭsakaḥ iti
Yuktaṃ çhaitaṭ, yatō jwarāatisāadayaḥ kāayaçhikiṭsāaviṣāaviṣayāa
rōgāa agnidōśāadēv bhavaṇti *(Ch. Su. 30/28 Shivdas sen)*

199. *Āayuṛbala ṣthitiriti aṇnapāaçhakāagni ṣthitāu*
āayuṛbala ṣthiṭyāa aṭyē5pyāatipṛēyāa vaṛṇāayō lakṣ́aṇēeyāaḥ *(Chakrapāaṇi)*
Aṇnapāanēṇdhanāiṣçhāagniṛjwalatiyaētipṛēyāa chāaṇyathāa *(Ch. Su. 27/342)*

unsettled bowels, diarrhoea, upward movement of abdominal wind, dropsy, dysentery and *Aphāra*[200].

b. *Teekshagni*

This is a very intense state of *jathrāgni* and causes swift and immediate digestion which leads to overeating. In this state it is also referred to as *Aṭyāgni* or *Bhaṣmak*. This state is a consequence of *Piṭta dosha* aggravation. The patient suffers from dryness of throat, lips and palate. He also feels a burning sensation and heat what areas after digestion of food.

c. *Manḍāgni*

This is the low intensity state of the *jathrāgni*. In this condition it becomes incapable of digesting even small amounts of food. This state is a consequence of *Kapha dosha* aggravation. The patient experiences heaviness in stomach and head, cough, asthma, increased salivation, vomiting and weakness[201].

d. *Samāagni*

When all the three *doshas –Vāta*, *Piṭta* and *Kapha-* are in balance, *jathrāgni* is also in balance and the food consumed in proper proportions is digested well. This state is called *Samāagni* (balanced *agni*). There is no abnormality in the digestive process in this state[202].

♦ *Bhūtāgnis*

This group of *agnis* is located in the liver. They are five in number according to the five elements they act upon:

1. *Bhaumāgni* (earth),
2. *Āapyāgni* (water),
3. *Āagniyāgni* (fire),
4. *Vāayavyāgni* (air) and
5. *Akāashāgni* (space)[203].

Each of these *agnis* transforms its

---

200. *Viṣamō dhāatuvāiṣamyaṃ karōti vi ṣamaṃ paçhaṇ*
Tēekṣ̣aṇō manḍēṇdhanō dhāatōoṇ viśoṣayati pāavakaḥ (Chi. Chi 15/50)
Yuktaṃ bhuktavatō yuḳtō dhāatusāaṃyaṃ samaṃpaçhaṇ
duṛbalō vidahaṭyaṇnaṃ taḍyāaṭyōoṛvamaḍhō5pi vāa (Ch. Chi 15/51)

201. *Aḍhaṣtu paẉamāamaṃ vāa p̣ravriṭṭaṃ grahaṇēegadaḥ*
Uçhyatē saṛvamēvāaṇnaṃ p̣rāayō ḥyaṣya vidaḥyatē (Ch. Chi 15/52)
Maṇḍāaṣṭēekṣ̣ṇō5tha viṣamaḥ samaśçhēti çhaturṛviḍhaḥ
Kaphapiṭṭāanilāadhiḳyāaṇjāaṭtaṭśāaṃyāaṇjāaṭtharō5nalaḥ (Ma. Ni. 6/1)

202. *Samāa samāagnēraśitāa māatrāa saṃyagvipaçhyatē*
Swalpā5pi nāiva maṇḍāagnē viṣamāagnēṣtu dēhinaḥ (Ma. Ni. 6/3)
Māaṭrāa5timāaṭmāa5pyaśitāa sukhaṃ yaṣya vipaçhyatē
Tēekṣ̣ṇāagririti taṃ viḍyāaṭ, samāagniḥ ṣ̣rēṣ̣thaḥ uçhyatē (Ma. Ni. 6/4)
Hitāaśēe ṣyāaṇnitāaṭ ṣyāalḳāalabhōjēe jitēṇḍriyaḥ
Paśyaṃ rōgāaṇ bahōoṇ kaśṭāaṇ buḍḍhimāaṇ viṣamāaśanāaṭ (Ch. Ni. 6/11)

203. *Bhāumāapyāagnēyavāayavyāaḥ paṇchōṣmāaṇaḥ sanāabhasāaḥ* (Ch. Chi 15/13)
Aṭra çha yāaṇyāaṇyaṇtarāaṇiupadhāatumalāadigatāani
tāaṇyavarōohāani bhōotāagniṣ̣vēva
Kiṇvāa, apradhāaṇyāadakiṇçhiṭkarāaṇi nōḳtāani (Charak)

corresponding element in the food broken down by *jathrāgni*, to match the state of body elements. Thus, these *bhūtāgnis* divide food into five parts which nourish the five elements found in different parts of the body.

♦ *Dhātvāgnis*

This is the third type of *agni* found in the body. When the *annaras* (digested food/ chyle), which has been transformed into five elements by the action of *jathrāgni* and *bhūtāgnis*, reaches the channels in the *dhātus*, it is further digested by the *Dhātvāgnis* located there. The *annaras* gets transformed into the seven *dhātus*. These are, hence, seven in number: 1. *Rasāgni*, 2. *Raķtāgni*, 3. *Māmsāgni*, 4. *Medāgni*, 5. *Asthi agni*, 6. *Majjāgni*, 7. *Shukrāagni* (in males)[204]. The action of these *agnis* not only regenerates the *dhātus* but also produces *malas* (waste products). When the *Dhātvāgnis* are aggravated, it leads to decrease in *dhātus*. Conversely, low intensity leads to increased *dhātus*.

The entire digestive process due to the action of the three types of *agnis* is explained here.

When food reaches the mouth, it is mixed with saliva and the taste is perceived. It then moves to the stomach where it turns watery, foamy, soft and smooth due to the action of the stomach juice which is liquid and oily. In this first step of digestion, foamy *kapha* and sweet *ras* are produced[205]. The digestion in the stomach during this stage can be likened to the boiling of rice in a utensil.

This half -digested *Ahāar-ras* reaches the intestines via duodenum. Here *jathrāgni* acts on it together with *Samvāyu* and *Pāchak pitta*[206]. *Pāchak pitta* absorbs the liquid, part of *Ahāar ras,* converting it into a solid mass which is referred to as '*pind*'. *Kātu Ras* and *Vāyu* are produced during this stage[207]. Food is segregated here into two parts: 1. *Sāar* and 2. *Asāar* or *kitt*.

The properly digested part which is in a liquid form is the *Sāar* part. This is the first

---

204. *Saptabhirdēhadhāatāarō dhāatavōdvividhaṃ puṇaḥ*
Yathāaswamagnibhiḥ pāakaṃ yāaṇti kiṭṭaprasāadavaṭ (Chi 15/15)

205. *Aṇnamāadāanakarmāa tu pṛāaṇaḥ koṣṭhaṃ prakarṣati*
taḍ ḍravāirbhiṇnasaṇghāataṃ ṣnēhēna mroditāaṃ gataṃ (Chi 15/6)
Aṇnaṣya bhuktamāatraṣya ṣaḍsaṣya prapāakataḥ
madhurāadyāaṭ kaphō bhāavāaṭ fēnabhōoṭ udēeṛyatē (Ch. Chi 15/9)
Madhuryāaṭ picçhhilaṭwāachcha praklēdiṭwāattathāiva cha
Āamāaśayē saṃbhavati ślēṣmāa madhuraśēetalaḥ (Su Sū 21/13)

206. *Aśitaṃ khāaditaṃ pēetaṃ lēeddaṃ koṣṭhagataṃ ṇriṇāaṃ*
Tajjēeryati yathāakāalaṃ śōṣitaṃ pittatējasāa (Su. Shā 4/19)
Paraṃ tu pachyamāanaṣya vidagdhaṣyāaṃlabhāavataḥ
Āaśayāachchyavamāanaṣya pittamachhamudēeryatē (Ch. Chi 15/10)

207. *Pakvāaśayaṃ tu parāaptaṣya śoṣyamāaṇaṇaṣya vaṇhināa*
Paripiṇdita pakvaṣya vāayuḥ syāaṭkaṭubhāavaṭaṭh (Ch. Chi 15/11)

of the *dhātus*- the *ras dhātu*- which is sweet and unctuous due to the action of *jathrāgni*. This *ras Dhātu* is then converted into other *dhātus*. If the *jathrāgni* is at low intensity, the *ras* turns bitter and sour. This is called the *āam* or *āamras*[208] which is toxic and disease-causing. That part of food, which is not digested properly, is called *asāar* or *kitt*. Its solid part changes to stool and liquid to urine, and collects in the bowels.

At this stage, the five *bhūtāgnis* join the metabolic process. They convert the form of the five elements in the digested food to match the form found in the body. This nourishes the earth element found in the body.

This *āhār-ras* is circulated around the body as *ras dhātu* through the *srotas* (body channels). This nourishing *ras*, in which are inherent the building blocks of all *dhātus*, thus reaches all the organs.

The digestive action of the *Dhātvāgnis* replenishes *dhātus* and produces *ojas*.

Piṭta plays a vital role in this entire digestive process. Hence several *Ayurved* experts do not differentiate between *Agnis* and *Piṭta*. It is true that the seven *Dhātvāgnis* contain parts of *Pāchak piṭta* that helps them function. But the *Agnis* also contain elements other than the *Piṭta*, and it is their combined action that completes the digestive process.

The *Ras* that is circulated around the body is acted upon by the seven *Dhātvāgnis* to create the seven *dhātus*. The *dhātus* are believed to have three parts, 1. *Sthōol* 2. *Sukshm* or *Anu* 3. *Mala*. The *Sthōol* part nourishes the *dhātu*, the *Sukshm* part creates the next *dhātu*, and the *mala* part forms the *mala* product. Hence, the action of every *Dhatvaagni* produces by-products and *mala*. For example, the *saar* (nourishing part of the food) is acted upon by the *sthōol* part of *ras Dhātvāgni* to create *ras dhātu*. The *sukshma* part of the same *dhātvāgni* creates the *rakṭ dhātu* and the *mala* part is converted to *Kapha* (phlegm, saliva, etc). The other *Dhātvāgnis* also act in a similar way.

S. No.	*Dhātvāgni*[209]	*Sukshm* (Nourishes)	*Sthōol* (Creates)	*Mala* (Waste products)
1.	*Ras*	*Ras Dhātu*	*Rakṭ Dhātu*	*Kapha* (phlegm, saliva)
2.	*Rakṭ*	Rakt Dhatu	*Mamsa Dhātu* (mixes with *mala*)	*Pitta (mixes with mala)*
3.	*Māṃsa*	*Māṃsa Dhātu*	*Med Dhātu*	Other *malas*
4.	*Med*	*Med Dhātu*	*Aṣthi Dhātu*	Sweat
5.	*Aṣthi*	Bones and Cartilage	*Majjā*	Hair and Nails
6.	*Majjā*	*Majjā Dhātu*	*Shukra*	Lustre in the eye and Unctuousness of skin
7.	*Shukra*	Sperm, Ovum		

♦ Āam Ras

When the *āhār ras* (nutritive part of the ingested food) is not properly digested due to decreased activity of *jathrāgni* or *dhātvāgnis*, it turns toxic and is called *Āamras*.The presence of *Āamras* in the body causes various ailments[210].The elements in the undigested *asaar* or *āamras* do not convert into a form acceptable to the body. Hence, the next step in the metabolic process of assimilation by *dhātus* and other body parts, does not occur. Being unable to move easily in the various body channels (*srotas*), it accumulates in different body parts like lung, heart and other organs. The four cavities that usually attract *āamras* are brain, chest, abdomen, and rectum, of which the abdomen is the most common site of *āamras* accumulation.

This leads to dyspepsia and other disorders. *Āamras* combines with *doshas* and attacks other organs causing various ailments like allergic asthma. When the low potency of *dhātvāgni* causes the formation of *āamras dhātu* (undigested), the next *dhātu*, i.e. the *rakṭ dhātu* is deprived of nourishment, again, leading to various ailments. Because almost all ailments are in one way or the other connected with the formation of *āamras*, they are sometimes also referred to as '*Amay*'.

Āamras affects the *agnis*, weakening the metabolic process and causing food to remain undigested. It also blocks the *srotas* (body channels). *Āam dosha* can occur in any part of the body. The weakest organs, and those with elemental composition similar to *āam dosha*, are most susceptible to its accumulation.

♦ Symptoms of *Sāam* Diseases

Blockage in the *srotas* (channels) of sweat,

---

208. *Sō5ṇnajō rasa iti āamaḥ*
Aṇnarasavyāivāapakavalya taṇtrāaṇtarē āamavyapadēśāaṭ (Madhukosh vyakhya)

209. *Rasāaḍraktaṃ tatō māaṃsa māaṃsāaṇmēdaṣtatōṣthi ̣cha*
Aṣtthnō majjāa tataḥ śukraṃ śukrāaḍ garbhaḥ praśāajaḥ (Ch. Chi 15/16)
Rasāatṣnaṇyaṃ tatō raktamasrijaḥ kaṇdarāaḥ sirāaḥ
Māaṃṣāaḍvasāa twaçhaḥ ṣaṭ ̣cha mēdasaḥ snāayusaṃbhavaḥ (Ch. Chi 15/17)
Pōoṛvō dhāatuḥ paraṃ kuṛyāaḍ ṿriḍḍaḥ kśēeṇaśçha taḍvidhaṃ (A. hr.)
Ṣthōolaśōokṣmamalāiḥ saṛvē bhidyaṇte dhāatavaṣtridhaa
Ṣwaḥ ṣthōolō5śaḥ paraḥ śōokṣmaṣtaṇmalaṃ yāati taṇmalaḥ (Su. Sū 14/10)(Dalhan)
Ṣwāagnibhiḥ paçhyamanēṣu malaḥ ṣaṭasu rasāadiṣu
Na śukṛē paçhgamāanē5pi hēmanēevāakṣyē malaḥ

210. *Āamāaśayaṣthaḥ kāayāagnēdāuṛbalyāaḍavipāaçhiṇtaḥ*
Āaḍya āahāara dhāatuṛyaḥ sa āam iti kēeṛtitaḥ (Madhukosh)
Āamasaṇnavarasaṃ kēçhiṭkēçhitu malasaṇchayaṃ
Pṛathamāaṃ dōśaḍriṣtiṃ ̣cha kē ̣chidāamaṃ pṛakśyātē (Madhukosh)
Avipakṿamasaṇyaktaṃ dugvaṇdhaṃ bahuviçhhilaṃ
Sadanaṃ saṛvagāatrāaṇāaṃ ḷtyabhidhēeyatē (Madhukosh)

urine, etc., weakness, heaviness, improper circulation of *Vāyu*, laziness, increased salivation and phlegm formation, absence of, or inadequate elimination of stool and other *malas*, apathy, fatigue, etc. are the symptoms of *sāam dosha* (*sāam* diseases). When characteristics opposite to the above mentioned symptoms are manifested, it is a sign of clean *srotas* and *nirāam dosha*[211].

As stated earlier, a weak digestive system causes the formation of *āam dosha*. When a *srota* is blocked by accumulation of either *āam dosha* or *mala*, the remedy is to increase release of the digestive juice in that *srota* in order to transform the *āam ras* into *dhātus*, or clearing away the *mala*. Therefore, most *ayuṛvedic* medicines contain substances that increase digestive power at some level. Purifying therapies such as *vamana* (induced nausea) and *virechan* (purgation), flush the *āamras*, *malas* etc. from the blocked *srotas*, clearing them and making the *agnis* more effective[212].

The potency of *Agnis* increases with age, resulting in strong and healthy digestive and metabolic activity. This nourishes the body, and boosts physical strength and growth. In a normal, healthy person, digestive power keeps gaining strength till the age of 40. Between 40-60 it remains steady. After 60 it begins to decline, preventing the body from getting all the nutrients that it needs. This leads to a deformation of *dhātus* and depletion in their numbers and strength. The body weakens and the quantity of *malas* increases. A person also experiences a draining of mental faculties. This is termed as old age. Rejuvenation therapies attempt to slow down this process of ageing and protect an individual from associated ailments by strengthening the various *agnis* (the complete digestive system)[213].

12. *Srota*

The word *srota* has been used very frequently in the preceding pages. It is clear by now that the clean and healthy *srotas* are necessary for a healthy body. *Srotas* are as important as the *doshas*, *malas* and *dhātus*.

What are *srotas* and their functions?

All body parts that are hollow (i.e. are dominated by the space element) carry

---

211. *Vāayurāamāaṇvayaḥ saṛtirāaḍhmāanakṛiḍasaṇçharaḥ* (*Charak*)
Āavilaṣtaṣtumāaṇṭyāabbnaḥ ṗratōpēe piçhhilaḥ kapha (*Charak*)
Uśmaṇō5lpabalaṭvēna dhāatumāahāamapāachitaṃ (*Charak*)
Duśṭamāamāaśyagataṃ rasamāamaṃ ṗraçhakṣatē
Aṇyē dōṣēḅhya aiva Tiduśṭēḅhyōśṇyamōoṛçhhanāaṭ (*Charak*)

212. *Pāachanai dēepanāiḥ ṣnēhāiṣṭāaṇ ṣwēdāiṣçha pariśḳṛitāaṇ*
Saṛvadēhaṗravijṛitāaṇ sāamāaṇ dośāaṇ niṛharēṭ (*Charak*)
Lēenāaṇ dhāatiśẉanuṭkilaṣṭāaṇ phalāadāamāaḍrisāaniva
Āaśṛamaṣya hi nāaśaya tē ṣyuṛduniṛharaṭwaṭa (*Charak*)

213. *Yajjarāavỵāadhiviḍhvaṇsi bhēṣajaṃ taḍ rasāayanaṃ* (*Shāaṛaṇgdhar*)

water, food, *malas*, *dhātus*, sound, nerve impulses etc. are called *srotas*. They also transport essential materials like *dhātus* from one part of the body to another.

These hollow body parts have different shapes and sizes. Some are tubes, others are long, thin and wide, and yet others have a system of branches, much like creepers. Some *srotas* are visible to the naked eye, while many others are not. They are the same colour as the substance they mainly carry[214].

♦ Functions of *Srotas*

Their main function is to transport food, plasma, blood and other *dhātus*, *doshas*, *malas*, life-force etc[215].

1. Transporting the nutritious food from the gastro-intestinal/enteral tract to the *dhātus* making it possible for them to regenerate.
2. Play an important role in cleansing the body by transporting wastes such as stool, urine, sweat etc. to their points of excretion.
3. Support life by sustaining breath.
4. No chemical element in the body can be nourished or suffer an increase or decrease without the help of the *srotas*.
5. Is central to all functions of the body, being responsible for all movements like transport of *malas*, communication of feelings, desires etc.

♦ *Srotas* and Origination of Diseases

The importance of *srotas* for the smooth functioning of body processes is evident. Consequently, it is of utmost importance that the *srotas* remain in their naturally healthy state, like the *doshas* and the *dhātus*. An unhealthy or diseased *srota* affects the surrounding *doshas* which cause ailments related to both. Healthy *srotas* enhance the smooth circulation of substances like *doshas* and *dhātus* throughout the body and speedy movement of *malas* to their excretory

---

214. *Āakāśēeyāavakāaśāanāaṃ dēhē nāamāani dēhināaṃ*
Sirāaḥ ṣṭrōtāaṇsi māaṛgāaḥ khaṃ dhamaṇyōnāaḍya
āaśayāaḥ *(Su. Shā 9/3 Dalhan)*
Ṣṭrōtaṇsi khalu pariṇāamamāapadyamāanāanāaṃ
dhāatōonāamabhivāahēeni bhavaṇṭyayanāaṛthēna *(Ch. Vi. 5/3)*
Mōolāaṭ khāadaṇtaraṃ dēhē ṗraṣritaṃ ṭwabhivāahi yaṭ
Ṣṭrotaṣtaditi vijgēyaṃ sirāadhamanivaṛjitaṃ *(Su. Sha 9/13)*
Ṣṭravaṇāaṭ ṣṭrotāaṇsill Mōolāaṭkhāadii ḥriḍyadiçhhiḍrāaṭ ṗraṣritam,
abhivahanaśēelaṃ, vadaṇtaraṃ avakāaśaḥ
Tat, sṭrōtō viggēyaṃ *(Dalhan)*

215. *Saṛvēhi bhāavāaḥ purōṣē nāaṇtarēṇa ṣṭrotāaṇṣyabhinir*
vaṛtaṇtē, kṣyaṃ vāadaṗyabhigaçhhaṇti *(Ch. Vi 5/3)*
Tadētaṭ ṣṭrōtasāaṃ ṗrakṛitibhōotavẏvāaṇna vikāarāirupa
-ṣrijyatē sarēeraṃ *(Ch. Vi 5/6)*
Ṣṭrōtasāa çha yathāaṣvēna dhāatuḥ, puśyati dhāatutaḥ *(Ch. Vhi 8/39)*

points[216]. Diseased *srotas* pass on their state of imbalance to the substances they carry, which in turn further corrupt the *srotas*. It becomes a vicious cycle. If a *dhātu* or *mala* accumulates in a *srota*, the metabolic process of that *dhātu* is hampered. The adjoining *srotas* are also adversely affected. This leads to *Āam Dosha,* which travels to other parts of the body polluting other *srotas* and causing ailments. Common cold and related diseases are a good example. Out of balance *dosha* travels from the diseased *nāsa srota* to the *srota* in the thoracic region causing cough. On reaching the ear it causes ear-ache, heaviness and deafness. It also causes sinusitis on reaching the head, tuberculosis in the lungs and dysentery on reaching the bowels. Hence it is crucial to keep all the *srotas* clean and in good health.

♦ Types of *Srotas*

Our body is a network of innumerable large and small *srotas*. Some like gastro-intestinal tract, arteries, veins, lymphatics, reproductive and urinary tracts etc. are visible to the naked eye. Others are so small that they can be seen only under the most powerful microscope[217].

---

216. *Tāani duṣṭāani rōgāaya viśudhāani sukhāaya çha* (A.H.Sha. 3/42)
Tē çhāavakāaśāaḥ prakupitāaḥ ṣthāanaṣthāaṇ māargaṣthōṣçha
dhāatōoṇ prakōpayanti Tēpi taṃ ṣtrotāasi çha
Ṣtrotāaṇśi dhāatavaṣçha dhāatōoṇ
Tēṣaaṃ saṛvēṣāamēva duṣisitāarō duṣṭāa dośāaḥ (A. San. Sha 6)
Āahāaraṣçha vihāaraṣçha yaḥ syāaḍdōśaguṇāiḥ samaḥ
Dhāatubhiṛviguṇaṣçhāapi ṣtrotaśāaṃ sa pradōoṣakaḥ (Ch. Vi 5/23)
Atipṛavṛitiḥ saṇgō vāa siṛāaṇāaṃ graṇthayō5pi vāa
Vimāargagamanaṃ çhāapi ṣtotasāaṃ duṣtilakṣ́naṃ (Ch. Vi 5/24)
Kupitāanāaṃ hi dōśāaṇāaṃ śarēerē paridhāavatāaṃ
Yaṭra saṇga khavāiguṇyāaḍ vyāadhiṣtaṭrōpajāayatē (Su. Sū 24/19)
Kṣipyamāaṇaḥ khavāiguṇyāaḍrasaḥ sajjati yaṭra saḥ
Karōti vikṛiti tatra khē vaṛṣamiva tōyadaḥ (Ch. Chi 15/37)
Pratirōgamiti kruḍḍhāa rōgāadhiṣṭhāanagāaminēeḥ
Rasāayanēeḥ prapaḍyāaśu ḏōśāadēhē vikuṛvatē (A. h. Ni. 1/23)

217. *Pṛāaṇōdakāaṇnarasarōdhiramāaṃsamēdōṣthimajjāaśukṛamōoṭra*
- Purēesaṣwēdavahāaṇēetiḥ
Vāatapiṭṭaślēṣmaṇāaṃ puṇaḥ saṛvaśarēeraçharāaṇāaṃ saṛvāaṇi
- ṣṭrōtāaṇsyayanabhōotāani
Taḍvaḍṭēeṇḍriyāaṇāaṃ punaḥ saṭvāadēenāaṃ kēvalaṃ
çhetanāavaçhharēeramayanabhootamadhiṣṭhāanabḥōotaṃcha (Ch. Vi 5/6)
Tathāa5paṛāaṇyaṇtaḥ ṣṭrōtaṇsi jēevitāathatanani
ṭrayōdaśa
pṛāaṇōbhāaṇnadhāatumalāanāamāayatanāani (A. San. Shā 6)

S. No.	Name and Function	Controlling Organ	Causes of Vitiation	Symptoms	Treatment
1.	*Prāṇa* Vahana *Srota* (Carries breath and Vitality)	Heart and Alimentary tract	Wasting, Suppression of natural ur ges, eating dry, ununctuous foods, exercising while hungry	Restricted hallow and rapid breathing. Asthma is related to this	Therapies for breathing problems
2.	*Udakvhar Srotas* (bears water and other liquids)	Palate, pancreas	Exposure to heat, indigestion, ingestion of excessive alcohol, eating extremely dry foods and remaining thirsty	Dry lips, tongue palate and throat	Treatment of excessive thirst
3.	*Aṇnavāha Srotas* (Carries food ingested from outside)	Stomach	Irregular eating habits, over-eating, unhealthy food and low digestive power	Appetite loss, vomiting, indigestion	Remedies for *āam* dosha and indigestion work well
4.	*Rasāvāha Srotas* (Carries chyle lymph, plasma)	Heart and the ten vessels connected with heart	Worry, diet comprising excessively heavy, cold and ununctuous foods	Anorexia, disguesia, ageusia, nausea heaviness, drowsiness, fainting, anaemia impotency	Fasting
5.	*Raktavāha Srotas* (Carries blood, especially Hemoglobin	Liver, spleen	Pungent, hot and oily food, exposure to excessive sun & heat	Chronic skin diseases, bleeding, abscesses, inflammation in anus and genital organs	Blood-letting
6.	*Māṃsavāha Srotas* (Carries ingredients of muscle tissue)	Tendons, ligaments and skin	Sleeping immediately after meal, frequent intake of heavy and gross foods	Granuloma, Myoma, piles, uvulitis, goiter, adenitis, tonsillitis cancers and non malignant growths	Surgery, heat therapy and *kṣhāra* therapy (local application of alkalis)
7.	*Medovāha Srotas* (Carries ingredients of fat tissue)	Kidneys, fat tissue in the abdomen	Sleeping during daytime, lack of exercise, excessive alcohol and oil-rich diet	Severe urinary disorders,	Weight reduction remedies

S. No.	Name and Function	Controlling Organ	Causes of Vitiation	Symptoms	Treatment
8.	*Aṣthivāha Srotas* (Carries nutrients of tissue)	Hip bone	Excessive exercise involving friction of bones intake of food that causes *Vāyu.*	Cracking nails and teeth, pain in bones, change in hair	Enema using herbal medication prepared with milk
9.	*Majjāvāha Srotas* (Carries nutrients of marrow)	Bones, Joints	Incompatible foods (fish and milk, honey in hot drinks etc.), injury to bone marrow by crushing, compression etc. of doshas on time	Pain in joints, giddiness, fainting, loss of memory, blackouts, deep abscesses	Using sweet and pungent substances, sexual activity, exercise treatment of excretion
10.	*Sukravāha Srotas* (Carries Semen Ovum & their nutrients)	Testicles, Ovary	Sex at improper time, unnatural sex, suppression or excess of sex	Impotency, infertility, abortion defective pregnancy	
11.	*Mūtravāha* Srotas (Carries urine)	Kidneys, Bladder	Food, drinks and sex during urge for micturition, suppression of the urge for micturition, specially by those suffering from Tuberculosis wasting.	Excessive quantities or no urine. Frequency of urination, thick urine.	Same treatment as for difficult urination
12.	*Vacrovāha/ Purisavāha Srotas* (Carries stool)	Colon, Rectum	Suppression of urge to pass stool. Taking food before digestion of previous meal. Weak digestion.	Less or excessive quantity of stool hard stool.	As for passing bowels
13.	*Svedavāha Srotas* (Carries sweat)	Fat tissue, hair-follicles	Excessive exercise, anger grief, fear, exposure to heat.	Absence of or excessive perspiration. Roughness of Skin. Horripilation (Hair erection). Burning sensation on skin.	As for fever

13. *Ātma*

What is *Ātma*?

The central principle of *ayuṛved* is — to maintain the health and harmony of the body[218]. The body is not merely a physical structure built by a combination of five elements and other chemical compounds. Body, and consequently Life, is a result of a union between the five elements, mind, intelligence and *ātma* (soul)[219].

Together with the five elements, the organs and the mind form the foundation of the body. The conscious part of this foundation is the *ātma*[220]. *Ātma* is considered to be the originator of all actions, as well as the bearer of their consequences. When the *ātma* leaves the body, the body becomes non-functional, or dead, even if all organs are intact. In the absence of the *ātma*, the organs cannot function, and nothing can be felt or experienced by the body. Hence, the *ātma* has been considered the basis of all consciousness[221].

The *ātma* is indestructible. It continues to live even after the body has been destroyed. It is immortal hence fundamentally different from the body. At the time of death it takes on another body according to the *karma* of the deceased body. Even though it is a conscious entity, it needs to enter into collaboration with intelligence, mind and sense organs in order to acquire knowledge, feel, communicate and be manifest[222]. It is when the *ātma* meets intelligence, that intelligence interacts with sense organs, and the organs absorb perceptions, that knowledge is gained[223].

♦ Characteristics of *Ātma*

Joy, sorrow, desires, hatred, effort, breathing, blinking of the eye, thought process, determination, memory, knowledge, inter-sensory communication, sound and other perceptions, motivation, beliefs, dreams, sexual desires, patience, pride – all these are considered qualities of the *ātma* because these characteristics are manisfested only as long as the *ātma* resides in the body and a person

---

218. *Ṣwaṣthaṣya śwāaṣṭhyarakṣ́ṇaṃ āaturaṣya vikāara ṗraśamaṇaṃ ċha* (Ch. Su. 30/26)
Eha khalụāayuṛveda ṗrayōjanaṃ vyāadhyupaṣriśṭāanāaṃ
vyaadhi parimokṣ́ah ṣwaṣthaṣya rakṣ́aṇaṇċha (Su. Sū 1/22)

219. *Śarēerēṇḍriya saṭwāaṭmasaṇyōgō dhāari jēeviṭaṃ*
Niṭyagaṣ́vāanubaṇdhaṣ́ċha paṛyāayāirāayuruċhyatē (Ch. Sū 1/42)

220. *Taṭrāayuṣ́chetanāanuvritiḥ* (Ch. Su. 30/22)

221. *Taṭra śarēeraṃ nāama chētanāadhiṣ́ṭhāanabhōotaṃ*
Paṇċhamahāabhōotavikāarasamudāayāaṭmakaṃ (Ch. Sh. 6/4)

222. *Āaṭmamaṇṣōḥ saṇyōgāviśeṣāaṭ saṇṣkāarāaċhċha ṣmritihi* (Vaiśēsikadarśan)
Āaṭmāa jgyaḥ karaṇāiṛyōgāajgyāanaṃṭwaṣya ṗravaṛtatē (9/2/6)
Karaṇāanāavāimalyāadayōgāaḍvaa na vaṛtatē (Ch. Shā 1/54)

223. *Manaḥpuraḥ sarāaṇiṇḍriyāaṇyaṛthagrahaṇaśamaṛthāani bhavaṇti*
Taṭra ċhakṣ́uḥ ṣ́rōṭraṃ grāaṇaṃ rasanaṃ spaṛśanamiti paṇchēṇdriyāaṇni (Charak Su. 8/7-8)

is alive. In fact, it is only with the existence of the *ātma* in the body, that sensory organs, mind etc. become functional. *Ātma* exists in the *drashta* or witness form[224]. A body can be treated only as long as the *ātma* resides in the body. No treatment works on a body that is bereft of the *ātma* and is referred to as dead[225].

14. Mind (*Māna*)

All organs of the body work in conjugation with the mind. No sensory organ can perceive knowledge without the support of the mind. Therefore, the mind is one of the most important parts of the human body[226]. It is considered both a sensory and a motor organ[227].

Āyurved, *Yog shāstrās* and other related books and treatises refer to the mind as '*mānas*'. It is made up of the '*mān*' *dhātu*.

---

224. *Prāaṇāapāanāu nimēṣāadyāa jēevaṇaṃ manasō gatiḥ*
Iṇdriyāaṇtarasaṇchāarah prēraṇaṃ dhāaraṇaṃ ċha yaṭ
Dēśāaṇtaragatiḥ swapnē paṇchatwagrahaṇaṃ tathāa
Driśtaṣya dakśiṇēnāakśṇāa savyēnāavagamaṣtathāa
Jeṿāa ḍwēṣaḥ sukhaṃ prayaṭnaśchētanāa dhritiḥ
Budhiḥ smritiraṇkāarō lingāani paramāatmanaḥ
Yaṣmāaṭ samupalabhyaṇtē liṇgāaṇyētāani jēevataḥ
Na mritaṣyāaṭmaliṇgāani taṣmāadāahumaharṣayaḥ
Śarēeraṃ hi gatē taṣmiṃ śōoṇyāagāaramachētanaṃ
Paṇchabhōotāa vaśēṣaṭwāaṭ paṇchatwaṃ gatamuchyatē (Ch. Shā 1/70-74)
Prāaṇāapāanāavuchhavāasaniḥ śwāasō (Chakrapāaṇi ch. Shāa)
- Ichhāaḍwēṣa prayaṭnasukhdukhdukhagyāanāaṇyaamāa nō liṇgaṃ iti (Nyāaya Parśan)
Prāaṇaa5nanimēṣōṇmēṣjēekaṇamanōgatēeṇdriyāaṇtaravikāarāḥ (1/1/10)
Sukha dukhēchhāa ḍwēṣa prayaṭnāaśwāaṭmanō liṇgāani (Vai. Da. 3/139)
Āaṭmāa jgyaḥ karaṇāiryōgāajgyāanaṃ ṭwaṣya pravartatē (Ch. Shā 1/54)
Taṭtwaṃ jalē vāa kaluṣē chētaṣyupahatē tathāa (Ch. Sha 1/55)

225. *Saṭtwamāaṭmāa śarēeraṃ cha trayamētaṭ tridaṇḍavaṭ*
Lōkaṣtiṣthati saṇyōgāaṭ tatra sarva pratiṣthitaṃ
Sa pumāaśchētanaṃ tacheha tachchāadhi karaṇaṃ smritaṃ
Vēdaṣyāasya tadartha hi vēdō5yaṃ saṃprakāaśitaḥ (Ch. Su. 1/46-47)

226. *Manaḥ puṇaḥ sarāaṇēeṇdriyāaṇyarthagrahaṇa samarthāani bhavaṇti* (Ch. Su 8/7)
Atikrāan,oṇdriyamaṭēeṇdriyaṃ chakśurāadēenāaṃ
Yadiṇdriyaṭwaṃ bāahyajgyāanakāaraṇaṭwaṃ, taḍ trikāaṇtāmityarthaḥ (Chakrapāani)

227. *Atēeṇdriyaṃ punarmaṇaḥ saṭwa saṇgyakaṃ chēta ityāahurēkē*
tadarthāatmasampaṭṭadāayaṭṭachēṣṭaṃ chēṣṭāa
pratyayayabhōotamitiṇdriyāaṇāaṃ (Ch. Su 8/4)

It is *'manas'* that is primarily responsible for any action or thought. Words like *chiṭta*, *ḥridaya* (heart), *swantah* etc. are all synonyms of *mānas*[228].

The mind is considered important because it is the crucial link between the *ātma* and the organs, whose interactions lead to acquisition of knowledge[229]. It is an unconscious entity and lacks colour, feelings and perceptions. But it is true that a body experiences all these only due to the interaction between the mind and the *ātma*. Every *ātma* has a mind, which is considered as its internal assistant and companion. Just as the sensory organs are the external means of collecting knowledge, mind is the internal means. It is one of the four main organs of the conscience.

According to the sages, *ātma* is the traveller/warrior, the body is the chariot, the intellect is the charioteer and the mind is the rein. The sensory organs are the horses, worldly affairs and subject matters are the different paths available. One who remains ignorant – who is unconscious, and has an intemperate and unregulated mind- loses control over his sensory organs which tend to behave like wild horses[230].

♦ Location

Mana is believed to reside in the heart and the brain. Both these organs are related to each other, and therefore they are dependent on each other. In *ayurvedic* texts, heart is considered to be the primary location of the *māna*, whereas the *yog* treatises consider both heart and brain equally important[231].

♦ Size And Number

According to *ayurved*, *māna* is atomic in size, is a single entity, and is a material[232].

♦ Functions

The main function of *mana* is to interpret sensory data collected by the sense organs and communicate it to the motor organs, brain and other sites of emotional and intellectual importance. As a result of this

---

228. *Maṇyatē avabuḍhyatē jgyāayatē anēna iti maṇahlmananāaṭ manaḥ*
Çhinṭanṭu çhētō ḥridayaṃ ṣwāanṭam, ḥriṇmāanasaṃ manaḥ **(Amarkosha)**

229. *Lakṣaṇaṃ manasō jgyāaṇṣyāabhāavō bhāava aiva c̄ha*
Sati ḥyāaṭmaṇḍriyāarthāanāaṃ saṇnikarṣē na vaṛtatē
Vāivṛityāaṇmaṇmaṇasō jgyāanaṃm sāaṇniḍhyāaṭṭaçhçha vaṛtatē **(Ch. Shā 1/18)**

230. *Aaṭmāanaṃ rathina viḍhi śarēeraṃ rathamēva tu*
Buddiṃ tu sāarthi viḍhi manaḥ pragrahamēna çha
Iṇḍṛiyāaṇi hayāanāahuḥ viṣayāanṭēṣu gōçharāaṇ
āaṭmēṇḍriya manōyukṭaṃ bhōkṭēṭyāahuṛmanēeṣiṇah
Yaṣṭwavijgyāanawāaṇa bhanaṭyayukṭēna manasāa sadāa
Teṣyēṇḍriyāaṇyava ṣ́yāani duṣṭāaṣ́vāa iva saarathēḥ **(Kathopaniśad 3/35)**

231. *Ṣaḍaṇgmaṇgaṃ vijgyāanamiṇhḍriyāanyaṛtha paṇchakaṃ*
āatmāaçha saguṇaṣ́çhētāaṣ́chinṭyaṃ ḥa ḥridi saṇṣ́ritaṃ **(Ch. Su 30/4)**

232. *Aṇuṭwamatha çhāikaṭwaṃ ḍwāu guṇāu manasaḥ ṣmritāu* **(Ch. Sha 1/19)**

process the motor organs are able to perceive outside information and react appropriately[233].

♦ Characteristics and Strengths

Like the three *doshas*, there are three types of '*mānas*' that are found in human beings:

1) *Satvā*

2) *Rājas*

3) *Tāmas*

The qualities of all three types can be discerned in every human being, but just like the *doshas* one or other type is predominant[234]. *Satvā* qualities constitute knowledge and light; *Rājas* constitute action; *Tāmas* represents senselessness and sloth.

Based on these qualities, mental powers are also divided into three types – *Sātvik*, *Rājsik* and *Tāmsik*. *Sātvik mana* is pure, ethical and conscious, *Rājsik mana* is restless and prone to anger, and *Tāmsik māna* is predominantly ignorant and unaware. Qualities of people with these *māna* characteristics are given below.

a. People with *Sātvik* characteristics

Rāajsik and *Tāamsik* characteristics are absent in such people. They have a high degree of consciousness, are forgiving, serene, pleasant, kind, simple, generous, detached, and have a clear heart and mind[235].

b. People with *Rājsik* characteristics

Such people are playful, capricious, proud, covetous, greedy, spiteful, sensuous, and have lust for intoxicants. They are often plagued by the consequences of their actions which are guided by these qualities[236].

c. People with *Tāṃsik* characteristics

They are ignorant, ill-informed, inert, lazy, lustful, meek, deluded, prone to attachment and heavy[237].

233. *Iṇḍriyāabhigrahaḥ kaṛma manasaḥ ṣwaṣya nigrahaḥ*
Ūhō viçhāarṣçha, tataḥ paraṃ buḍḍhiḥ pravaṛtātē (Ch. Sha 1/21)
Iṇḍriyēṇēṇḍroyāarthō hi samanṣkēna graḥyatē
--- dośatō5thavāa (Ch.-Sha 1/22)

234. *Taṭ (Sawaṃ) ṭrividhamāakḥyāayatē - śuḍḍhaṃ, rāajasaṃ, tāamasaṃmiti* (Ch. Sha. 3/13)
Yaḍguṇaṃ çhāabhēekṣṇaṃ puruṣamanuvaṛtatē saṭwaṃ
taṭsaṭwamēvōpadiśaṇti munayō baahulyāanuśayāaṭ (Ch. S4 8/6)

235. *Sāatṿikāastu-āaṇriśasyaṃ saṃvibhāagu ruchitāa titikṣśāa*
Saṭyaṃ dhṛma āaṣtikyaṃ gyānaṃ buddhiṛmēdhāa ṣmritiṛḍhritirana
- bhiṣaṇgṣçha (Su. Sha 1/23)

236. *Rāajasāaṣtu - dukha bahukatāa5tanaśēelatāa5ḍhritirahaṇkāara*
Āaṇritiķriṭwamākāarōoṇyaṃ daṃbhō māanō haṛṣaḥ kāamaḥ ķrōdhāṣçha (Su. Sha 1/24)

237. *Tāamasāaṣtu - viṣāadiṭwaṃ nāaṣtikyamadharma śeelatāa*
Buddhēṛnirōdhō5jgyāanaṃ duṛmēdhaṣṭwakaṛmaśeelatāa
niḍrāaluṭwaṃ çhēti (Su. Sha. 1/25)

Decrease or increase in the quantity of these characteristics results in the three types of personalities.

♦ *Mana* and *Āyuṛved*

It is an established fact that the qualities and condition of the mind and body affect each other. Therefore, in the *āyuṛvedic* system of medicine, both the physical and the mental condition of the patient are taken into consideration before a treatment is finalized. *Āyuṛved* divides ailments into two categories – 1) physical 2) mental/ psychological[238].

The causes of the physical ailments are disturbances in the body, whereas the mental ailments are caused due to disturbances in the mind or '*mana*'. But it is realized in *Ayuṛved* that *mana* also contributes to the physical ailments. Bodily functions and physiological processes are controlled by the '*māna*'. Conversely, mental processes are affected by physiological conditions. This deep relationship between the two is the rationale behind treating physical ailments using therapies for mental health and well-being.

238. *Śarēeraṃ saṭṭwa sanjgaṃ ċha vyāadhināamāaśrayō matahḥ* *(Ch. Su 1/55)*

Matter – Introduction

The previous chapter dealt with various components and elements that sustain the body, like *doshas*, *dhātus*, *malas*, *srotas*, etc. Health and holistic well-being is a matter of balance and harmony amongst all the constituent elements. Whenever there is a drop or an increase in the quantity of these elements, balance is restored by the consumption of food or other curative substances with similar or opposing qualities. How does one determine what substances share the qualities of a particular *dosha* or *dhātu*, or what foods and herbs can correct a *dosha* or *dhātu* vitiation? This is possible only with an in-depth knowledge about all aspects of matter/ substances.

All things in the universe are principally made up of the five elements[239]. Like the *doshas* and *dhātus*, all substances are also created by a combination of the five elements in differing quantities. The shape and colour does not indicate the predominant element of any substance. Only an awareness of the taste essence (*ras)*, post-digestive taste/ bio-transformation (*vipaka*), potency (*vīṛya*) and other properties (*gunas*) will help identify the chief element of any substance. Based on this knowledge, a therapist chooses the most appropriate food and medicinal substances for a particular patient.

Medicinal substances are divided into many categories. The three main ones are:[240]

a. ***Pāarthiv Ḍravya*:** Substances found on and in the earth are known as *Pāarthiv* substances. Soil, sand, metals (like iron, copper, gold, silver, etc.), mercury, pearls, gemstones, pieces of clay vessels etc. fall under this category[241].

b. ***Jaaṇgam Ḍraṿya*:** This includes all medicinal substances obtained from the animal world. Leather, blood, meat, animal fat, bones, bone marrow, sperm, milk, hair, nails, fur, horns, teeth, feathers, sinew, hooves, abdominal organs, uterus, bile etc[242].

c. ***Āuḍbhid Draṿya*:**[243] This category includes plants and all substances obtained from them. Different kinds of flora, fruits, flowers, roots, seeds, leaves, branches, *bark*, plant exudates, gums etc. are all categorized under *Āuḍbhid dravya.*

Based on the constituent elements,

---

239. *Saṛvaṃ ḍravyaṃ pāaṇçhabhāutikamaṣminṇaṛthē* *(Ch. Sh 26/10)*

240. *Taṭpunaṣṭriviḍhaṃ jgyēyaṃ jāaṇgamāuḍbhidapāaṛthivaṃ* *(Ch. Su 1/69)*

241. *Suvaṛnasamalāaḥ paṇçhalōhāaḥ sasikatāaḥ sudhāa*
Manaḥśilāalē maṃayō lavaṇaṃ gāirikāanjanē *(Ch. Su. 1/71)*

242. *Madhōoni gōrasāaḥ piṭṭaṃ vasāa majjāa5ṣrigāamiṣaṃ* *(Ch. Sū 1/69)*
Viṇmōoṭra çhaṛmarētō5ṣthi ṣṇāayuṣringāaḥ ḳhurāaḥ
Jaṇgamēḅjyaḥ p̣rayūjgaṇtē kēśāa lōmāani rāçhanāaḥ *(Ch. Su. 1/70)*

243. *Uḍbhiḍya p̣rithiviṃ jāayatē iti āuḍḅhidaṃ ṿrikśāadi* *(Ch. Da.)*

substances are also divided into five categories. Its important to remember, that all substances have traces of all five elements. Most substances are dependent on earth and water which play a role in their formation. The three remaining elements – fire, air, space - complete the process of creation and add to the uniqueness of each substance. But every substance has a dominant element that decides its properties and makes it unique. On the basis of this fact, the five types of substances are:

1. *Pāarthiv ḍrav̤ya* (earth)
2. *Jaliēy ḍrav̤ya* (water)
3. *Vāyavya ḍrav̤ya* (air)
4. *Tejas ḍrav̤ya* (fire)
5. *Āakāŝhiya ḍrav̤ya* (space)

Characteristics of each of the above are listed in the previous chapter.

According to *ayuṛved*, the taste essence or *ras* of a substance is the most important characteristic that needs to be looked into during substance analysis. Hence, we will first discuss about *ras*.

1. *Ras* (Taste)

Ras is that property which helps determine the dominant element of any substance. How does one identify the *ras* of a substance? This is a skill acquired with great practice. Just as touch on skin helps us to understand texture, touch on the tongue helps us to understand taste[244]. What is the effect of taste on the physiology of a person? This also helps determine the *ras* of a substance.

There are six kinds of basic tastes[245] – sweet, sour, salty, pungent, bitter and astringent. Sweet provides the highest amount of energy. The potency decreases as one travels down the list. Thus, astringent taste provides the least amount of energy.

Ras and the Five Elements

Though sweetness is the natural property of water, it is produced only after an interaction with the other elements. Similarly, each *ras* has a predominant element[246].

---

244. *Rasēṇḍriyāagrāaḥyō yō5ṛthaḥ sa rasaḥ* *(Shi)*
Raṣyatē āaṣāaḍyatē iti rasaḥ *(Ch. Do)*
Rasanāaṛthō rasaṣtaṣya *(Ch. Sū 1/64)*

245. *Ṣwāaduraṃlō5tha lavaṇaḥ kaṭukaṣtiḳta aiva ç̣ha*
Kaṣāayaśç̣hēti ṣaṭkō5yaṃ rasāanaaṃ saṇgraḥ ṣaṇritaḥ *(Ch. Su. 1/65)*

246. *Tēṣaaṃ ṣaṇṇaaṃ rasāanāaṃ sōmaguṇāatirēkāaṇmadhurō rasaḥ*
p̣rithiv̤yagnibhōoyēṣ̄thaṭwāadaṃlaḥ, salilāagnibhōoyēṣ̄thaṭwāalḷavaṇaḥ
Vāay̤vagnibhōoyēṣ̄thaṭwāaṭ kaṭukaḥ, vāay̤vāakāaśaatiriḳtaṭwāaṭṭiḳtaḥ
Pavanp̣rithuvēev̤yatirēkāaṭkaṣāaya iti *(Ch. Su 26/40)*
Ḳṣ̣māa5ṃbhō5gnikṣ̣māaṃbutējaḥ khavāay̤vagṇyanilagō5nilāiḥ
ḍwayōvṇāiḥ ḳramāaḍḍhōotāiṛmadhurāadirasōḍbhavaḥ *(A.h. Su 10/1)*

	(1)	(2)	(3)	(4)	(5)	(6)
RAS	Sweet	Sour	Salty	Bitter	Pungent	Astringent
ELEMENT	Earth Water	Water Fire	Air fire	Air Fire	Air Space	Air Earth

The effect of any substance on an individual *dhātus, doshas*, etc. depends on the main element of the *ras*.

Although there are six primary tastes, they combine in several ways to form innumerable taste variations. Apart from these, there are other taste types that are not immediately clear, but manifest themselves faintly after a while[247].

Ras and *Doshas*

Depending on its dominant element, a *ras* will increase or decrease the potency of a *dosha*. For eg[248].

Ras	Increases	Decreases
Sweet	*Kapha*	*Vāyu, Piṭta*
Salty	*Kapha, Piṭta*	*Vāyu*
Sour	*Piṭta, Kapha*	*Vāyu*
Bitter	*Piṭta, Vāyu*	*Kapha*
Pungent	*Vāyu*	*Piṭta, Kapha*
Astringent	*Vāyu*	*Piṭta, Kapha*

Ras and *Dhātu*

Six primary *ras* types and *dhātus* are also intimately related. Normally:

Sweet, Sour, Saline *rasas*	–	increase the quantity of *dhātu*;
Bitter, Pungent, Astringent *rasas*	–	decrease the quantity of *dhātus*;
Pungent *rasas*	–	decrease in *med*, *majjā* and *lasika*
Sour *ras*	–	decreases in *Shukra*

247. *Tatra yō ṿyakṭaḥ sa rasaḥ,*
Yaṣthi raśēnāabhibhōotaṭwāaṇna ṿyajyatē ṿyajyatē vāa kiṇehidaṇtē so5nuraśaḥ (*Yo*)

248. *Swāadwaṃlalavaṇāa vāayuṃ, ḳaṣāayaṣwāadutiḳtakāaḥ*
Jayaṇti piṭtaṃ, śtēṣmāaṇaṃ kaṣāayakaṭutiḳtakāaḥ (*Ch. Su. 1/66*)

249. *Kaṭwaṃlalavaṇaaṃ vāiḍyēvidāahina iti ṣṃritāaḥ* (*R. Vai. bhā*)
ṣwāadutiḳtakaṣāayāaḥ ṣbhuvidāaharahitāa rasāaḥ

Ras And Mala		
Sweet, Sour, Saline *rasas*	–	Help in excretion of waste products (hence helps during constipation)
Bitter, Pungent, Astringent *ras*	–	Helps retain waste products (hence beneficial during diahorrea)

Two Classes Of *Rasas* :

Based on digestive patterns, *rasas* are divided into two types – *vidaahi* (causing extreme thirst, heart burn) and *avidaahi* (causing no burning sensation during digestion, relieves exhaustion)[249].

Vidaahi	–	bitter, sour and salty taste
Avidāhi	–	sweet, pungent and astringent taste

Identifying *Ras* and Their Qualities (*Gunas*)

Sweet Taste

That which produces certain amount of stickiness on chewing, nourishes body[250], clears sense organs, is preferred by ants, is the sweet taste.

This *ras* and products containing this *ras* (medicines and food products) are useful; they nourish and boost the quantities and strength of all *dhātus*, and increase life-span. Such substances improve complexion and provide strength. Intake of sweet *ras*-rich substances eases aggravated *Pitta* and *Vāyu doshas*, and neutralizes the adverse effects of toxins. They lend strength, beauty, flexibility and stability to the body. They make the nose, throat, mouth, tongue and lips soft. Sweet substances are unctuous, cool, and heavy. They are good for hair, sense organs and *ojas*, and they help increase milk production. Therefore, thin people, children and recovering patients must increase intake of sweet foods.

Despite its beneficial qualities, excess of sweet taste can cause an increase in the *Kapha dosha*. As a result ailments like obesity, laziness, excessive sleep, lack of appetite, weak digestion, diabetes, accumulation of fat around

250. *Taṭramadhurōrasaḥ śarēera sāaṭṃyāaḍrasarudhira maaṃsa*
mēdō5ṣthimajjāujaḥ
Śuḳrāabhivaṛdhana āayuśyaḥ ṣadinḍriyapṛaśāadanō balavaṛṇa karaḥ
Piṭlaviṣamāarutaghnaṣṭriśṇāadāaha praśamanaṣṭwaçhyaḥ kēśyaḥkanṭhayōbalyaḥ
Pṛēeṇanōjēevanaṣtaṛpaṇōḅriṇhaṇaḥ ṣthāiṛyakaraṇ
Ḳśēeṇakṣnatasaṇdhāanakarō
Gṛāaṇamakhakaṇthānṣthajivyāapraḥlāadanēe dāahamōoçhhāa praśamanaḥ
Ṣaṭpadaṛpipēelikāanāamiṣtatamaḥ ṣnigdhaḥ śeetō guruṣçha (Ch.Su 26/42)

Taṭrayaḥ paritōṣamuṭpāadamati, pṛaḥlāadayati, taṛpayati, jēevayati,
muktōpalēpaṇjanayati, ślēṣmaaṇaṃchāabhivaṛdhayati samadhuraḥ (Su. Su 42/11)

neck and face, urinary problems, cough, cold, fever with cold, sweetish taste in the mouth, lack of sensation, weak voice, goiter, enlarged cervical glands, swelling of throat, stickiness in throat, conjunctivitis, are easily contracted[251]. Therefore obese and overweight people, diabetics and those having stomach worms must refrain from consuming sweet foods.

Sweet foods/ substances : *Ghēe* (clarified butter), milk, sugarcane, jagery, walnut, banana, coconut, falsa, shatavari, kakoli, jack fruit.

Exceptions : Old rice, old barley, wheat, green gram, honey, [Abutilon indicum or (Kanghi in Hindi), *Sida spinosa/ Grewia hirsuta (Nagbla)*, Meda, Maha Meda, *Desmodim gongeticum* (Sarivan-Hindi), Daterdime seeds *(Uraria Picta)*, *Vigna trilobata* (Mungran in Hindi), Ban Black gram (Wild gram) *(Mashparni)*, Leptadenia reticulate (dori in Hindi) *(Jivanti)*, Malaxis muscifera *(Jivak)*, Butter Tree *(Mahua)*, Liquorice Root *(Mulaithi)*, Indian Kudji *(Vidari)*, Thorny Bomboo *(Vanshlochan)*, Gmeling arborea *(Gambhari)*, Gokhru, Grapes, These are all sweet items, even though sweet, do not cause *kapha* vitiation.]

♦ Sour Taste

The taste that causes the mouth to water, brows to contract, and teeth the /gums to tingle, is the sour taste.

It adds to taste and makes food interesting. It boosts appetite and is cool to touch. Sour foods/ substances nourish the body and toughen it, make the brain more active, fortify and strengthen the heart, strengthen the sense organs, and energize the body. The juices of such food substances help in boosting digestion by adding moisture and softening it. Sour foods are refreshing, light (easy to digest), smooth and warm. They aid waste elimination. Unripe fruits generally have sour taste.

Consumption of too many sour foods/ substances increases *piṭta* in the body and symptoms like excessive thirst, horripilation, teeth disorders, melting of *kapha*, damaged muscles, body-swelling in thin people, weakness, feebleness, lowering of body temperature, itching, darkness before the eyes, dizziness, skin diseases, pus formation in cuts and wounds, burning sensation in throat, heart and chest[252]. Therefore people suffering from skin diseases, stress, asthma, cough, sore throat, pain in the joints should avoid sour

---

251. *Aṃlōrasō bhakṭaṃ rōçhayati, agnidēepayati, dēhaṃ ḅriṇhayati,*
Ūṛjayati
manōbōdhayati. inḍṛiyāaṇiḍṛuḍēekarōti, balaṃvaṛdhayati,
Vāatamanulōmayati *(Ch. Su 26/42)*
Yo daṇtahaṛṣamuṭpāadayati, mukhāasāaṃ vajanayati,
Ṣ́ṣraḍdhāaṃ çhōṭpāadayati, so5ṃlaḥ *(Su. Su. 47/11)*

252. *Daṇtaaṇ haṛṣayati, taṛṣayati, saṃmēelayoṭyakṣ́ēeṇēe, saṇvējayati lōmāani*
Kaphaṃ vilāapayati, piṭtamabhivaṛdhayati, rakṭaṃ dōoṣayati,
māaṃsa vidahati,
Kāayaṃ śithilēekarōti, kṣ́ēeṇakṣ́takṛiśaduṛbalāanāaṃ
ṣwayathumāadayati *(Ch. Su. 26/42)*

foods. Thin people, and those whose diet lacks oily/unctuous items, should eat very little sour foods.

Exception: Pomegranate and dried pomegranate seeds, Indian gooseberry *(amla)*, Tamarind *(Imli)*, lemon, silver, mango, *Kamzakh, Karonda & Kaith.*

Curd and Buttermilk though sour are not harmful.

♦ Salty Taste

The taste that causes salivation and burning sensation in throat and cheeks is the salty taste.

Saline foods carry *vāyu* downwards, aid digestion, enhance taste, create stickiness and are pungent. They reduce stiffness in joints, accumulation of fat, waste products and blockade in *srotas*[253]. Saline foods are not oily, hot or heavy. This taste essence reduces the potency of other essences.

Excessive salinity vitiates both the *piṭta dosha* and the blood, leading to increased thirst and heat sensitivity. It causes burning sensation, dizziness, decrease in blood and other *dhātus*, rotting of infected skin (if suffering from skin diseases), mouth ulcer *(mukhpak)*, eye ulcer *(netrapak)*, swelling, discolouration of skin, bleeding, weakening of gums, increased toxicity, decreased virility, baldness, graying of hair, wrinkles, erysipelas, ringworm, hyperacidity, gout, increase in time of wound healing and reduction of strength and *ojas*[254]. Salt is considered unwholesome for the eyes. Hence, salt should not be taken by patients of skin diseases and high blood pressure.

♦ **Salty foods/substances:** Rock-salt, *saurvachal namak*, black pepper, sea salt, *salt* produced from earth, *Audbhid namak.*

Exceptions: Rock salt doesnot cause any harm.

♦ Bitter Taste

This taste agitates the front part of the tongue, causes watering of eyes, nose and mouth, and burning in the cheeks.

Bitter substances purify the mouth, aid absorption of food, boost hunger and digestion. They clean and improve the efficiency of sense organs, remove waste products from eyes, nose and *srotas* more

---

253. *Pāachanaḥ kḷēdanō dēepanaṣ̣chayāvanaṣ̣chhēdanō bhēdanṣ̣ṭēekṣ̣ṇaḥ*
Sarōvikāaṣyadhaḥ
Ṣraṇṣyavakāaśakarō vāataharaḥ ṣtaṃbhabaṇdhasaṇghāatavidhamanaḥ
Saṛvarasapṛaṭyanēekabhōotaḥ *(Ch. Su. 26/42)*
Lavaṇaḥ saṇśōdhanaḥ pāachanō viśaṇāa kḷēdanaḥśāithiḷgakṛiduṣṇaḥ
Saṛvarasapṛatyanēekō māaṛgaviśōdhaṇaḥ saṛrvaśarēerāavayavamāaṛ
-davakaraṣ̣cheti *(Su. Sū 42/14)*

254. *Sa aivaṃ guṇō5śyēka aivāaṭyaṛthumupayhjyamāanaḥ piṭṭaṃ*
kōpayati, rakṭaṃ vaṛdhayati, taṛṣayati, mōoṛchhayati, tāapayati
dāarayati, kṛiśṇāati māaṃsāani pragāalayati kuśṭhāani *(Ch. Su 26/42)*
Sa aivaṃ gaṇō5pyēka aivāaṭyaṛthamāasēvyamāanō gāaṭra
Kaṇdōokōthaśōphavāivaṛṇya
Puṇṣṭwōpaghāatēṇḍrajvōpatāapamukhāakṣipāakarakṭa
Piṭṭavāatāśōṇitāaṃlikāa pṛabhritināapāadayati *(Su. Sū 42/14)*

effectively. Hence, bitter foods help in keeping the *srotas* of *anna, ras* and blood clear. Bitter taste helps cure obesity, hives, conjunctivitis, eye fatigue, itching, sores, worms, stiffness of joints, throat infections, leprosy etc. It dries oil, *med*, *māṃsa* and *ḳled*. It calms *kapha* and circulates sluggish blood. It also adds variety to taste[255].

Excess of bitter taste leads to dizziness, anxiety, dryness of lips and palate, fatigue, asthma, weakness, fainting, reduced virility and decrease in sperm count. Being dominated by air and fire elements, excessive intake leads to burning in limbs and back, fever, body ache, stinging and smarting pain, and other deformities[256].

♦ **Bitter foods/ substances:** Asafoetida, false pepper, black pepper, (Indian long pepper and its root), cinnamon, white leadwort, ginger, ink nut, all kinds of *piṭta*, urine and marking nut *(Bhilawa)*.

♦ **Exceptions:** Dry ginger, long pepper and garlic are safe bitter taste foods and do not cause any harm.

♦ Pungent Taste

This is the taste that removes stickiness from the mouth and numbs the tongue.

Despite tasting bad, the pungent taste essence enhances taste of other substances adding variety to food. Pungent foods detoxify, and help cure stomach worms, leprosy, itching, fainting, burning sensation, thirst, skin diseases and fever. They aid circulation of *vāyu* and create dryness. Consequently they help in drying up moisture, fat, obesity, bone-marrow, lymph, pus, sweat, urine and stool. They purify the throat and the liver and increase efficiency. Fever and toxins caused by accumulation of *āam* are effectively purged. They purify breast milk and calm *Piṭta* and *Kapha doshas*. This taste essence is light, dry, cool and smooth, and is excellent for intelligence[257].

Excessive intake of this taste essence causes a reduction in plasma, blood, fat, bone marrow and sperm count. It also leads to roughening of the walls of the *srotas*, drying of the mouth, reduction of strength, thinness, fatigue,

255. *Kaṭukō rasō vaḳṭraṃ śoḍhayati, agniṃ dēepayati, bhuḳtaṇ5ōayati,*
ghrāaṇamāaṣrāavayati, çhaḳṣ̣urvirēchayati, ṣphutēekarōtēe
-ṇḍriyāaṇi, rōçhayaṭyaśanaṃ, kaṇḍōoṛvināaśayati, ṿriṇāaṇvasāa
- dayati, ḳrimēeṇ hinaṣti *(Ch. Sū 26/42)*
Kaṭukōdēepanaḥ pāachanōrōchanaḥśōdhanaḥ ṣthāulyāalaṣyakapha
-Ḳrimiviṣakuṣ́thakandōo ṗraśamanaḥ
Saṇḍhibaṇḍhaviçhhēdanō5vasāadanaḥ ṣtaṇyaśuḳramēdasāamu
-pahantāa çheti *(Su. Sū 42/05)*

256. *Puṇṣṭwamupahaṇti, rasavēerya ṗrabhāavāaṇmōhayati, glāapayati*
kanthaṇparidahati
śarēeratāapamupajanayati, balaṇḳṣ́iṇōti, ṭriṣ́ṇāaṇjanayati *(Ch. Su. 26/42)*
Sa aivaṃguṇō5pyēka aivāaṭyaṛthamupasēṿyamāanō ḅhṛa̱mamadagalatāa
-lụōṣ́thōṣ́ōṣadāahasaṇtāapabalanighāatakaṃpatōḍbhēdaḳriṭ
Karçharaṇāapāaṛṣ́va ṗriṣ́tha ṗraḅhritiṣu çha vāataśoolāanāadayati *(Su. Sū 42/15)*

dizziness, fainting, and *vātaj* ailments like torticolis, facial paralysis, headache, pain[258].

♦ **Pungent foods/substances:** Jute (*Patoli*), Sandalwood, *khuś* (the grass *andropogon muraticum*), *Swertia Chirata (chirayta)*, nēem, tinospora (*giloy*), wild gourd, sweet-flag, khorasan thorn *(Dhamasa), Maha Panchmul* Medicine Ayurvedic, small and big *kateni,* Bitter cucumber, Atecs, vach.

♦ **Exceptions:** *Giloy* and *patoli* though pungent are not harmful.

♦ Astringent Taste

The Astringent taste essence numbs the tongue and blocks the throat and the *srotas*.

This taste essence destroys *Piṭta* and *Kapha doshas*, controls blood pressure, helps heal wounds, aids healing of broken bones, dries *medak*, liquid *dhātus*, urine etc., causes cessation of stool during dysentry and dissolves fat. Intake of astringent foods causes constipation and hardening of the body. They make the skin excessively soft and cause wounds and boil and increase stress on diseased and infirm parts. Astringent taste foods are dry, cool and heavy[259].

Excessive intake of astringent foods leads to dryness in mouth, heartache, bloating of the stomach, speech impediment, blocking and shrinking of *srotas*, darkening of complexion, reduction of virility, excessive thirst, weakness, hardness and decline of *vāyu* (*adhovāyu*), obstruction in the smooth movement of urine, stool, other waste products and sperm. Because astringent foods are heavy, their digestion takes a longer time. Because these foods aggravate *Vāyu*, their intake might in some cases lead to

---

257. *Tikṭōrasō ṣwayamarōchiṣṇurapyarōçhakaghnōviṣaghnaḥ ḳrimighnō Mōoṛçhhāadāahakaṇdōokuśṭhaṭriṣṛāa praśamana ṣṭwaṇmāaṃsayōḥ Ṣthirēekaraṇō* *(Ch. Sū 26/42)*
Tikṭāṣçhhēdanō rōchanōdēepanaḥśodhanaḥ kaṇdōokuśṭhatriṣṇāa -mōoṛçhhāajwara praśamanaḥ ṣṭaṇyaśodhanō Viṇmōotraḳlēdamēdōvasāa pōoyōpaśoṣaṇaṣçheti *(Su. Sū 42/16)*

258. *Rāukṣyāaṭḳharaviśadaswabhāavāaçha rasarudhirmāaṃsamēdō5ṣthi -majjaśukraanyuçhhōṣaśayati* *(Ch. Su. 26/42)*
Gāaṭramaṇyāaṣṭaṃbhāakṣepa kāarditaśirahṣoolabhramatōḍ -bhedaçhchhēdāasyavairaṣyāanyāapāadayati *(Su. Sū 42/16)*

259. *Kaṣāayō rasaḥ saṅśamanaḥ saṅgrāahēe saṇdhāankaraḥ pēedanōrōpaṇaḥ śoṣaṇaḥ ṣṭambhanaḥ Ślēṣmaraḳtapiṭta praśamahaḥ śarēeraḳlēdaṣyōpayōḳtāa rōoksaḥ Śeetō5laghuṣcha* *(Ch. Sū 26/43)*
Kaṣāayaḥ ṣaṅgrāahakōpaṇaḥ ṣṭambharaḥ śodhanōlēkhanaḥ Śōṣaṇaḥ pēedanaḥ ḳlēdōpasōṣaṇaṣçheti *(Su. Sū 42/16)*

260. *Āaṣyaṇ5ōṣayati, ḥridayaṇpēedayati, vdaramāadhmāapayati, vāachaṇnigriḥṇāati, ṣrōtāaṇṣyavabaḍhṇāati* *(Ch. Su. 26/43)*
Ḥriṭpēedāa5ṣyaśōdarāaḍhmāanavāakyagrahamaṇyāaṣṭaṃbha -gāaṭraṣphuraṇaçhumuçhumāayanāayanāakuṇchanāakṣēpaṇa prabhritēenjanayati *(Su. Sū 42/17)*

an attack of palsy, paralysis, stiffness and convulsions[260].

♦ **Astringent foods Stat:** Myrobalan *(harad)*, Belliric Myrobalan *(bahedā)*, *Albizzia Lebbek (shrish)*, Cutch Tree (Katha tree in Hindi) *(khair)*, honey, *Anthocephalus Cadamba (kadaṃb)*, *Ficus glomerata* (Country fig) *(gular)*, raw caveat, lobis stem pearls; coral *(praval)* and gern are astringent substances.

♦ **Exceptions:** Even though Myrobalan *(harad)* is astringent, it is not cool and does not obstruct stool elimination etc.

The qualities of all foods and herbs depend on their taste essence. Medicinal preparations are more potent and this potency also depends on the taste essence of the ingredients. For example taste essence medicines are cold, and sour or bitter medicines are hot.

2. Attributes

All substances have different attributes and hence their effect on the body varies. *Ayuṛved* describes 20 such attributes that are found in 10 opposing pairs:[261]

1. Heavy	2. Light
3. Dull	4. Sharp
5. Oily, Greasy	6. Dry
7. Cold	8. Hot
9. Smooth (Guṃmy)	10. Rough
11. Solid	12. Liquid
13. Soft	14. Hard
15. Subtle	16. Bulky
17. Stable	18. Fluid
19. Non- (Tremulous) mucilaginous	20. Mucilaginous

These attributes are not physical but medicinal. These qualities depend on the effects the substances have on the body[262]. Just because a substance feels heavy on holding does not mean that it has the heavy attributes. Heaviness and lightness depends on the time taken to digest it. That which is easily digested is light and that which takes time to digest is

261. *Gurulaghuśēetōṣṇaśnigḍharōokṣaṇdatēekṣṇaṣthirasaraṃridu -kathinviśada piçhhilaślaķṣṇakharaṣthōolasōokṣmāsāaṇdra ḏravāaḥ viṣatiḥ*

262. *Kaṛmbhiṣṭwanumēeyaṇtē nāanāaḍravyāaṣrayaaḥ guṇaaḥ* (Su. Sū 46/513)

heavy. Similarly linseed that feels cold is actually hot because it increases the temperature in the blood and *taste* essence.

These attributes also depend on the proportion of the five elements they contain. If earth is the dominant element, it is heavy; if sky dominates, it is light. As stated earlier, only the taste essence cannot help to determine the attributes, they can be judged on the basis of both taste and effects on the constitution.

3. *Virya*-Potency

All medicines have a combination of many attributes out of which one or two dominate and are capable of curing ailments. These attributes determine the potency of the medicine[263]. Potency is more powerful than taste essence. Medicines are divided into two types based on their potency – *cold* and *hot*. This is what is popularly known as the hot or cold quality of a substance. Hot or cold medicines are prescribed according to the nature of the ailments. It is the potency that cures ailments and boosts health. During digestion the physical and curative chemical composition of the medicine changes. This affects the *doshas* and the *dhātus*. Based on these effects sweet, pungent, and astringent substances are classified as cold and sour, salty and bitter substances as hot.

♦ **Effects on the body**

Cold potency substances[264] cool the body and lend moisture. Using these substances leads to increase in age, *dhātus* (especially semen) and life strength. Hence they can be used as tonics. They calm *Piṭta* and increase *Vāyu* and *Kapha*.

Hot potency substances[265] increase heat in the body. They also increase digestive power, sweat, thirst, and thinness. They calm *Vāyu* and *Kapha* and aggravate *Piṭta*.

Some experts also consider six other potencies in addition to these two while deciding the attributes of any medicine. They are – 1. Unctuous 2. Dry (Unctuous) 3. Heavy, 4, light 5. Dull 6. Sharp. It can thus be said that there are 8 potencies[266], but the two main ones are the hot and the cold potencies.

When the potency is weak it is referred to as merely an attribute. There are some medicines which do not have potency. While foods have taste essence, medicines have potencies.

---

263. *Vēeṛyaṃ tū kriyatē yēn yāa ḳriyāa* (Ch. Sū 26/65)

264. *Śeetaṣya ḍraḥdāadanaviśyaṇdana ṣtharēekaraṇaprasāadana -ḳlēdanajēevanāani* (Su Sū 41/11)
Śeetaṇḥlāadanaṣtaṃbhanajēevanaraḳtapiṭtapraśaadanāadēeni (A.S. Su 17/16)

265. *Taṭra kaṛmāaṇyaśyuṣṇaṣya dahanapāachanamōoṛçhhanaṣwēdana -vamanavirēchanāani vśṇaṣnigahāu vāataghnāu* (Su Sū 41/11)

266. *Mridutēekṣṇagurulaghuṣnigdharōokṣōṣṇa Śeetalaṃ Vēeṛyamśtavidhaṇkēchiṭ* (Ch. Su 26/64)

4. *Vipak* After Taste

The taste essences produced after the action of the initial stages of digestion, are called *Vipak*[267]. During digestion, a substance interacts with several digestive juices that alter it completely. During this entire process it passes through three phases. In the first phase its taste essence is sweet, in the second it is sour and in the third it becomes bitter.

In the last stages of digestion the nutritive and the waste parts of a substance are separated. After this the substance is nothing but its taste essence. It is different from the original taste essence and is called the *vipak.*

Types of *Vipak*

Based on the taste essence there are three kinds of *vipak* (after tastes) – sweet, sour and bitter. Sweet and salty substances have sweet *vipak,* sour substances have sour *vipak*, and pungent, bitter and astringent substances have bitter *vipak*[268]. Some exceptions are seen to the above stated types eg:

Substance	taste essence	*vipak*
Oil	sweet	bitter
A type of salt *(Sauvarchal)*	salty	bitter
Gooseberry (*Āmlā*)	sour	sweet
Dry ginger *(Shunthi),* Long Pepper-*Pippali*	bitter	sweet
Chebulic Myrobalan *(Haritaki)*	astringent	sweet
Trichosanthes dioica *(Patol)*	pungent	sweet

Effects Of *Vipak*: Effects of *vipak* depend on the taste essence.

Sweet *Vipak*: Purifies urine and stool and strengthens *Kapha* and semen[269].

Sour *Vipak*: Light, purifies urine and stool, weakens semen and strengthens *pitta*[270].

---

267. *Jāatharēṇāagninīāa yōgāadyadudēti rasāantaraṃ*
Rasāanāaṃ pariṇāamāaṇtē sa vipāaka iti ṣmritaḥ (Va.Sū 9)
Rasāanāaṃ pariṇāamāaṇtē jaraṇaniṣṭhāakāalē
Yaḍraśāantaraṃ rasaviśeṣaḥ udēti utpadyatē sa vipāakaḥ (A.D.)

268. *Katṇtikṭa kaśāayāaṇāaṃ vipāakaḥ pṛāayaśaḥ kaṭuḥ*
Aṃlō5ṃlaṃ paçhyatē ṣwāadurmadhuraṃ lavaṇaṣtatha (Ch. Su. 26/58)

269. *Madhuraḥ ṣriṣṭavinṃōotrō vipāakaḥ kaphaśukṛalaḥ* (Ch. Su 26/61)

270. *Piṭtakriṭ sriṣṭavinṃōoṭraḥ pāakō5mlaḥ śukṛanāaśanaḥ* (Ch. Sū 26/62)

5. *Prabhāv* (Specific Action)

Based on the above given details it seems that medicines act according to their taste essence (*ras*), potency (*vīṛya*) and after taste (*vipak*). It is not true always. Some substance matters have their own specific effect on the body which could be beneficial or harmful according to the ailment. The property that determines this effect is called *prabhāv*[271]. In other words, the different and unique effects produced by two substances on the body even after having the same *ras, vīṛya* and *vipak,* is termed as its *prabhāv*. Therefore, despite having similar *ras, vīṛya* and *vipak,* one medicine might be curative for a particular illness while another might aggravate it eg. – Both Purging Cotton *(jamālghotā)* and leadwort *(chiṭrak)* have bitter *ras* and *vipak*, and are hot, yet both cause motions Both Liquorice root *(mulāithi)* and Grape *(drākṣhā)* have the same *ras, vīṛya* and *vipak*, yet Liquorice root *(mulāithi)* is vomit inducing while Grape *(drākṣhā)* is not. *Ghēe* and milk also have the same properties but only *ghēe* is a digestive substance.

There are some medicines that need not be ingested. Merely tying or wearing them cures ailments (fever, insomnia, etc.). for example - tying the root of Purple/Ash-colored fleabane *(sahadevi)*on the head cures fever. Charms, gemstones, chants etc also heal due to the *prabhav* in them.

Medicines are divided into three categories based on their *prabhāv*:

1. *Shāman* (destroying) medicines: those ting) medicines: those that aggravate *doshas* and *dhātus*.
2. *Swasthyahitkari* (nourishing) medicines: those that provide nourishment.

Therefore to understand medicines and their effects on the body, one must be able to understand their *ras*, *vīṛya*, *vipak* and *prabhāv*. The strongest trait among them dominates and weakens the others. Hence, *vipak* is stronger than *ras* because it overshadows it; *vīṛya* is more powerful than both *ras* and *vipak* as it negates both of them. *Ras* is the weakest and *prabhāv* the strongest. In order of power they can be arranged as follows:

Ras – vipak – viṛya – prabhāv

6. Types of Medicine/Substances According To Effects

Guided by their *ras*, *vipak*, *vīṛya* and *prabhāv*, medicines affect the body. On the basis of the effects produced, they can be classified as:

---

271. *Rasavēerya vipāakāanāaṃ sāamāaṇyaṃ yaṭra lakśyatē*
Viśēṣaḥ kaṛmaṇāaṃ çhaina prabhāavaṣtaṣya sa ṣmritaḥ (Ch. Su 26/67)
Rasāadisāaṃyē yaṭ kaṛma viśēesṭaṃ taṭ prabhāavajaṃ
Daṇtēe rasāa dhāiṣtulyāa5pi chiṭrakaṣyavirēchanō (A.hr. Su. 9/26)

Vāman	They induce vomiting and help eliminate *kapha* and *piṭta* through the mouth[272]. *Mantal* is an example.
Virechan	Increase stool, help transport and excrete wastes[273]. eg.- Indian Jalap *(trivrit)*, *kāarśhikā* fruit etc.
Sanghrahi	That which binds stool or causes constipation.[274] eg. – cumin seeds
Brihan	Provides nourishment. eg. – (Hookex stocks) new *(guggul)*
Lekhān	Helps eliminate *dhatus* and *malas*-(Hookex stocks) (old *Guggul)*.[275]
Pachan	Digests undigested food, (without increasing digestive power). eg. - *Mesua ferrea* (Mesua)[276]
Shaman	Calm aggravated *doshas*. eg. – Tinospora *(giloy)*[277]
Anuloman	Helps gas trapped in the stomach to descend. eg. - Myrobalan *(harad)* [278]
Sansan	Helps to excrete hard stool, relieves constipation. eg. - *Amaltāas* [279]
Bhedan	Helps eliminate both hard and *dwaroop* stool from. eg. - *kuṭkī* [280]
Çhhedan	Forcefully eliminates hardened accumulated *doshas*. eg. – water and honey [281]

272. *Apakavaṃ piṭtaślēṣmāaṇnaṃ balāadōoṛdhavaṃ nayēṭtu yaṭ*
Vamanaṃ tadhi vijgēya madanaṣya phalaṃ yathāa *(Bhaa, Ora. Pōoraa Misra 6/219)*

273. *Vipakwaṃ yadapakwaṃvāa malāadi ḍravatāaṃ nayēṭ*
Rēçhayaṭyāapi tajgyēyaṃ rēçhanaṃ ṭrivṛitāa yathāa *(Shaarangdhar 4/7)*

274. *Ģrāahi taçhçha yathāa śunthēe jēerakaṃ gajapippalēe* *(Shaarangdhar 4/12)*

275. *Ḍhāahōoṇmalāaṇ vāa dēhaṣyaviśeṣṭejōḷḷekhayēçhça yaṭ lēkhanaṃ* *(Shaarangdhar 4/11)*

276. *Paçhaṭyāamaṃ na baḥviṃ çha kuṛyāadyaṭṭāḍvi pāaçhanaṃ* *(Shaarangdhar 4/2)*

277. *Na śodhayati na ḍwēṣṭi samāaṇḍōśāaṇstathōḍdhatāan*
Samēekaroti viṣamāaṇśamanaṃ taḍyathāaṃritāa *(Shaarangdhar 4/3)*

278. *Ķriṭwāa pāakaṃmalāanāaṇyaḍbhiṭwāa baṇdhamadhōnayēṭ*
Taçhçhāanulomaṇaṃ jgyēa yathāa pṛoktāa harēetaki *(Shaarangdhar 4/4)*

279. *Paktavyaṃ yaḍpakṭvāiva śliṣṭaṃ koṣthē malāadikaṃ* *(Shaarangdhar 4/5)*
Nayaṭyadhaḥ ssroṇsanaṃ taḍyathāa ṣyāaṭakritamāalakaḥ

280. *Malāadikamabaḍḍhaṃ yaḍbaḍḍhaṃ vāa piṇditaṃ malāiḥ*
Bhiṭwāa5ḍhaḥ pāttayati yaḍbhēdanaṃ kaṭukēe yathāa *(dŏ Po 4/6)*

281. *Śliṣṭāaṇkaphāadikāaṇ dōśāanuṇmōolayati yaḍvalāaṭ*
Çhhēdanaṃ taḍyathāa kṣāarāa māariçhāani śilāajatu *(dŏ Po 4/10)*

Grāhi	Strengthens *dēepan* and digestion, and relieves constipation. eg. – cumin seeds[282]
Stambhan	Stops oozing and removal, easily digestible and being astringent they cure constipation. eg. - *Vatsak*[282]
Rasāayan	Cures old-age ailments, increases life-span. Eg. – gooseberry, Hookex stocks *(guggul)*[283]
Vaajikar	Aphrodisiac. eg. – milk, *uḍad* pulse, asparagus *(shataavri)*, Liquorice root *(mulāithī)*[284]
Shukral	Increases quantity of semen. eg. – Winter Cherry *(aṣ̌hwagandha)*, mooslee, sugar, asparagus *(shataavri)* [285]
Sukshm	Those that can enter the body through pores. eg. – rock salt, honey[286]
Vỵāvāayi	Those that spread in the body before being digested. eg. Marijūana. [287]
Vikāshi	Calming the limbs and ligaments at the joints. eg. – betel-nut[288]
Prāmaathi	Removing accumulated *doshas* in *srotas* (body channels). eg. – black Pepper[289]
Abhiṣ̌hyaṇdi	Blocking *srotas* and causing heaviness due to their gravity and unctuousness. eg. – curd[290]

---

282. *Rāukṣ̌yāaçhhāityāaṭkaṣāayaṭwāalạlaghupāakāaçhçha yaḍbhavēṭ*
Vāatakṛiṭṣṭṃhanaṃ taṣyāaḍyathāa vaṭsakaṭuṇṭukāu *(Shaarangdhar P 4/13)*

283. *Rasāayaṇaṃ çha tajyēyaṃ yajjarāavỵāadhināaśanaṃ*
Yathāa aṃritāarudaṇtēe çha guggulaṣ̌çha harēetakēe *(dŏ Po 4/14)*

284. *Yaṣmāaḍ ḍravỵāaḍbhavēṣtrēesu harṣō vāajēekaraṃ çha taṭ* *(Shaarangdhar 4/15)*

285. *Yaṣmāaçhhukṛaṣya vṛidhi ṣyāaçhhukṛalaṃ hi taduçhyatē*
Yathāa5śvagaṇdha muśalēe śaṛkarāa çha śatāavarēe *(Shaarangdhar 4/16)*

286. *Dēhaṣya śūkṣ̌maçhhidrēṣu viśḍyaṭsūkṣ̌mamuçhyatē*
Taḍyathaa sāindhavaṃ kṣ̌āuḍraṃ niṃbatāilaṃ rūbōoḍụhbhavaṃ *(Shaarangdhar Po. 4/19)*

287. *Pōoṛva vỵāapỵāakḥilaṃ kạayaṃ tatah̤ pāakaṃçha gaçhhati*
Vỵavāayi taḍyathāa bhaṇgāa fēnṃ çhāahisamuḍbhavaṃ *(Shaarangdhar Po. 4/20)*

288. *Saṇdhibaṇdhāaṇṣtu sithilāaṇyaṭkarōti vikāaśi taṭ*
Viṣ̌ṭēśyāujaṣ̌çha dhāatibḥyō yathāa kramukoḍravā *(Shaarangdhar Po. 4/21)*

289. *Nijavēeṛyēṇa yaḍ ḍravyaṃ ṣrōtobḥyō dōśa saṇchayaṃ*
Nirasyati pramaathi ṣyāaṭṭṭyathāa marichaṃ vachāa *(Shaarangdhar Po. 4/24)*

290. *Pāiçhhilyāaḍ gāuravāaḍ ḍravyaṃ ruḍḍhavāa rasavahāah̤sirāah̤*

Health Horizons

The primary aim of *Ayurved* is to protect health and prevent diseases[291]. Maintenance of health depends on the condition of the *tridoshas* in the body[292]. It has been stated earlier that the *doshas* have a natural tendency to increase/decrease and be aggravated depending on the different time of the day and different seasons. Hence, to maintain the balance of the *tridoshas* through the day and the year, *Ayurved* prescribes health and life style rules suited to the season and the time of the day[293] which has two categories: *Dincharya-* (behaviour patterns and food habits during the day and night time)- and *Ritucharya-* (seasonal patterns and habits). A life style modelled on these precepts not only maintains health, it protects against the onslaught of diseases.

1. Dincharya

♦ Rising[294]

A healthy person must get up two hours before sunrise. This hour is considered auspicious as there is peace, freshness and happiness all around. The first act should be to think of God and pray. This creates mental peace and joy, because this is an hour when the mind and the heart are fresh, and whatever is thought, is remembered. Rising early also gives adequate time for ablutions and other routine activities, which in turn ensure a disease free and long life. Planning out the day's routine before leaving the bed ensures that all work is completed successfully on time.

♦ Washing Face

Washing face with fresh cool water immediately after leaving bed cleans dirt of the eyes, nose, mouth and face, and relieves early morning dullness. In winters luke warm water can be used[295].

---

291. *Ṗrayōjanaṃ ċhāaṣya ṣwaṣthaṣya ṣwāaṣṭhyarakṡaṇamāaturaṣya*
Vikāarapṛaśamaṇaṃ ċha
(Ch. Sū 30/26)
Iha ḳhalẉāayuṛvēela ṗrayōjanaṃ-vyāaḍhyupṣriṣṭāanāaṃ
Ṿyāadhi parimokṡhaḥ, ṣwaṣthaṣya rakṡaṇaṃ ċha
(Su. Sa 1/13)

292. *Dōśa dhāatumala mōolaṃ hi śarēeraṃ*
(Su. Sū 15/3)

293. *Māanavō yēna vidhināa ṣwaṣthaṣtiṣṭhati saṛvadāa*
Tamēva kāarayēḍvāidhō yataḥ ṣwāaṣṭhyaṃ sadēṗsitaṃ
Dinaċhaṛyāaṃ niśāaċhaṛyāaṃriṭuċharyāa yathōditāaṃ
Āaraċhaṇ puruṣaḥ ṣwaṣthaḥ sadāa tiṣṭhati nāaṇyathāa
(Bhā. Pra. Po. 5/12-13)

294. *Ḅrahṃē muhuṛtē uṭtiṣṭhējjēeṛṇāa5jēeṛṇa nirupaẏaṇ*
(A.S. Sū 3/3)
Dhaṭṭē yaḍgāuravaṃ taṭṣyāadabhiṣyaṇdi yathaa dadhi
(Sharangdhar Po. 4/25)

♦ Water intake on an empty stomach

At least one and upto four glasses of water should be taken after washing the face in the morning. Water should preferably be stored in a copper container at night. Drinking this cool water in the morning is beneficial. It helps in smooth and regular elimination of urine and stool in the morning, which is absolutely essential for removal of toxins from the body and protection from ailments.

Some people prefer drinking tea instead of cold water for the purpose of cleaning the bowels. Tea, being a hot and stimulating liquid, mimics the effects of water, by exciting the bowels and causing expulsion of wastes. But there is a subtle difference. The effect of tea on the bowels wanes after some time and the person begins to suffer from constipation. Also, the '*caffeine*' in coffee and tea harms the stomach and intestines. Water, on the other hand, has no side/ill-effects. Only people suffering from cold, cough and sore throat should warm the water before drinking.

♦ Ablutions[296]

Early morning clearing of bowels is a must after taking water . Modern-day busy and stressful living causes many people to suffer from lack of bowel movement in the morning. Indigestion, lack of sleep, stress, anger, depression, imbalanced personality can all lead to this problem. Eating food (heavy pulses, fried foods) that cause gas formation obstructs stool movement in the intestines. As a consequence, after only a little elimination, one feels that the bowels have been cleared. Later, one feels the need to repeat the process. Some people have to visit the toilet 3-4 times every morning.

Early morning rush to reach the workplace on time also contributes to the problem. People do not devote sufficient time to this activity. This leads to loss of appetite, gas, indigestion, headache, depression, self-pity, restlessness, fatigue, laziness, insomnia etc. Too much gas formation pressurizes the heart leading to an increased rate of heartbeat. Prolonged suffering from gas leads to serious

---

295. *Ṣpriṣṭvāa dhāatōoṇ naalāaṇaṣru vasāakēśanakhāaṇṣçhyutāaṇ*
Ṣnāaṭwāa bhōḳtumanāa bhuḳṭwāa ṣuptwāa ḳ ṣuṭwa surāaṛchanē
Raṭhyāamāaḳraṃya çhāaçhāamēdupuiṣṭa udaṇmukhaḥ
Ṛraṇmukhō vāa viḳtiṣthō na bahiṛjāanu nāaṇyahaḳ
Ajaḷpaṇnuṭṭarāasaṇga ṣwaçhhāiṛaṇgaṣṭamōolagāiḥ
Nōḍdhatāirnāanatō nōṛḍhvaṃ nāagnipaḳwāiṛna pōotibhiḥ
Na fēnabuḷbuḍḳṣāarāirnāi kahaṣṭāaṛpitāiṛjatāiḥ
Nāaṛḍrāika pāaṇiṛnāamēḍhyahḍyahaṣtapāadō na śaḅdavaṭ (*A. S.Sū 3/9-12*)

296. *Jāatavēgaḥ samuṭṣrijēṭ*
Udaṇmukhō mōotraśaḳriḍdaḳśiṇāabhimukhō niśi
Vāachaṃ niyaṃya ṛrayataḥ saṇvēetāaṇgō5vaguṇthitaḥ
Ṛravaṛtayēṭ ṛrachalitāṃ na tu yaṭnāadudēerayēeṭ (*A.S.Su. 3/3-4*)

ailments like chronic cold, asthma, piles, joint pain and arthritis. It is hence essential to clear bowels every morning. Eating heavy foods (heavy pulses, fried foods) should be avoided. Intake of green leafy vegetables, green gourd, and fibre-rich foods should be increased. If one feels the need to clear bowels more than once, it should not be avoided.

♦ Cleaning Teeth

1. Teeth should be cleaned with twigs (*dātōon*) that have bitter, pungent or astringent qualities because they protect the mouth from oral diseases. Twigs with sweet, sour and saline taste essence aggravate *kapha* and should be avoided. The best teeth cleaners are *Nēem* and *Babōol* twigs[297].
2. The twig (*dātōon*) should be carefully selected. It should be 6 inches long so that it can be held firmly and the tongue can be cleaned. It should be as thick as the little finger. A thicker twig will injure the gums. The front end of the twig should be soft (not dry and hard) so that it can easily be fashioned into a brush with a little chewing. It should be straight and not twisted[298].
3. The movement of the twig (*dātōon*) over each tooth should be from top to bottom and vice versa. This cleans the teeth thoroughly and does not damage the gums. Tooth powder can also be used simultaneously. This morning activity cleans the teeth, tongue and mouth; it keeps bad breath in check and stimulates the taste buds[299].

Various kinds of tooth brushes and tooth pastes are available in the market and are used more than naturally available twigs[300].

---

297. *Vaṭāasanāarkakhadirakaranjakaravēerajaṃ*
Sarjāarimēdāayapāargamaalatēe kakubhōḍhavaṃ
kaṣāaya tiktakaṭukaṃ mōolamaṇyadapēeḍriśaṃ
Vijgyāatavṛikṣaṃ kṣuṇnāagramrijwagraṇthi subhōomijaṃ (A.S.Sū 3/13-14-15)
Niṃbaśçha tiktē śrēṣṭhaṃ ķaṣaayē khadiraṣtathāa
Madhōokō madhurē ṣrēṣṭhaṃ karaṇjaḥ kaṭukē tathāa (Suṣrut Ch. 24/6)
Karaṇjakaravēerāarkamāalatēekakubhāasanāaḥ
Sasyaṇtē daṇtapawanē yē çhāapyēvaṇvidhāa ḍrumāaḥ (Ch. Sū 5/73)

298. *Tatrāadāu daṇtapawanaṃ ḍwāadaśāangulamāayaṭaṃ*
Kamiṣṭhikāa parēeṇāahaṃrijwagraṇthitaṃ vriṇaṃ (Sū Ch. 24/4)
Kanēeṇyagrasmaṣthānlayaṃ sukōorçhçhaṃ ḍwāadaśāangalaṃ (A. S.Su. 3/115)

299. *Daṇtāaṇ pōorkamadhō gharṣēṭ prāataḥ simçhēçhdia lōchanē*
Tyapōorṇamukhō grēeṣmaśaradōḥ śēetavāariṇāa (A. S. Sū 3/23)

300. *Nihaṇti gaṇdhaṃ vāiraṣyaṃ jivḥāa dhṇtāasyajaṃ malaṃ*
Niśķraśya ruchimāadhaṭtē sadyō d daṇtaviśodhanaṃ (Ch. Sū 5/72)
Tathāaṣya malavāiraṣyagaṇdhṇdhāajiṿhāa55ṣyadaṇtajāaḥ
Ruchivāiśadyalaghutāa na bhavaṇti bhavaṇti cha (A.S. Sū 3/18)

The tongue should be cleaned after the teeth, as food gets deposited on its surface. If not cleaned regularly, it gives out a foul smell and also obstructs taste perception[301]. The twig used to brush teeth can be used to clean the tongue. Tongue scrapers made of wood, silver, brass, copper, steel etc.,[302] that are available in the market, can also be used. The scrapers should be smooth and flexible. The edges should not be sharp or pointed as they might cause injury to the tongue.

It has been suggested that cleaning of teeth with a twig (*dātōon*) should be avoided if suffering from indigestion, nausea, asthma, fever, paralysis, excessive thirst, mouth ulcer (*mukhpāk*) and ailments of the heart, eyes, head and ear as there is a possibility of aggravation of disease if twigs are used under such conditions[303].

♦ Gargling[304]

If for some reasons teeth cannot be cleaned in the morning, gargling with water will help. It cleans the teeth, the tongue and refreshes the mouth to some extent. It also removes stickiness of the mouth and *kapha* accumulated in the throat and mouth. Ideally, after brushing the teeth, the mouth should be cleaned with sesame or mustard oil. (This process is called *kavalgṛah*). This strengthens

---

301. *Lēekhēḍanusukhaṃ jiṿhāaṃ jiṿhāanirḷēkhanēna ċha* *(A.S. Sū 3/17)*

302. *Jiṿhāanirḷēkhanaṃ rāuṗyaṃ sāuvaṛṇa vāaṛkṣamēva ċha*
Taṇmalāapaharaṃ śaṣtaṃ ṃriduślakṣṇaṃ daśāaṇgulaṃ *(Such. 24/13)*
Suvaṛṇarupyatāaṃṛāaṇi ṭrapurētimayāani cha
Jiṿhāanirḷēkhanāani ṣyuratēekṣṇāanyaṇrijōoni cha
Jiṿhāamōolagataṃ yaċhċha malamuċhhwāasarōdhi ċha
Dāuṛgaṇḍnyaṃ bhajatē tēna taṣmāsjiṿhāaṃ viniṛlikhēṭ *(Ch. Su. 5/74-75)*

303. *Nāadyāadjēeṛṇavamathuśwāaṣkāasajwaṛāaṛditēe*
Ṭṛṣṇāaṣyapāakaḥrinnetṛaśirahkaṛṇāamayēe ċha taṭ *(A. S.Su 3/19)*
Na khāadēḍ galatāalyōṣtha jiṿhāarōg samuḍbhavē
Athāaṣya pāakē śwāasē cha kāasahikkāavamēeṣu ċha
Duṛbalōśjēeṛṇabhakṭaśċha mōoṛċhhāaṛtāu madapēeditaḥ
Sirōrōojāarṭtaṣiṣtaḥ ṣṛāanṭaḥ, pāakakḷamāaṇvitaṃ
Aṛditēe kaṛṇaśōolēe c̄ha daṇtarōgēe c̄ha māanavaḥ *(Su. Chi 24/10-12)*

304. *Mukhavāiraṣya dāuṛasyadāurgaṇḍhya śophajāadyaharaṃ sutham*
Daṇtadāaṛḍyakarṃ rōoċhyaṃ snehagaṇḍōoṣadhāaraṇaṃ *(Su. Ch. 24/14)*
Haṇvōṛbalaṃ ṣwaṛbalaṃ vadanōpaċhayaḥ paraḥ
ṣyāaṭparaṃ ċha rasajgyāaṃṇuē ċha rōoċhiruṭtamāa
Na ċhāaṣya kaṇthaśōṣa ṣyāaṇnāuṣtahayōḥ sphuṭanāaḍbhayaṃ
Na ċha daṇtāaḥ ḳṣyaṃ yāaṇti riḍmōotāa bhavaṇti cha
Na śōotyaṇtē na ċhāamlēna ṇriśyaṇtē bhakśyaṇti cha
Parāanapi kharāaṇ bhakṣyāaṇṣtailagaṇḍōoṣaḍhāaṛaṇāaṭ *(Su. Chi 5/78-80)*
ōṣṭhṣphuṭanapāaruśyamukha śōṣaḍvijōomayāaḥ
Na ṣyuḥ ṣwarōpaghāatāaśċha ṣnēhagaṇḍōoṣadhāaraṇāaṭ *(A. S. Su. 3/29-30)*

teeth and gums, prevents toothache, reduces excessive sensitivity to hot, cold and sour substances (that sometimes cause toothache), improves voice quality, smoothes skin on face, and boosts taste perception and appetite. Regular rinsing of the mouth, gargling and *kavalgrah* prevents drying of throat and chapping of lips.

Substances with bitter essence boiled in water are excellent for gargling. Gargling and *kavalgrah* should be done in a wind-free and sunny spot. Mouth should be filled with the medicinal preparation, which should be held till mouth is filled with *kapha*, or *kapha* secretion takes place from the eyes and nose. When the quantity of the concoction prevents it from being moved in the mouth, the process is referred to as '*gandōśh*'. When the liquid can be moved around, the process is called '*kaval*'. *Kaval* helps to treat ailments of head and ear, laziness, indifference, chronic cold, nausea etc.

♦ The Head

The head should be oiled daily with sesame or coconut oil. This prevents hair fall, greying, balding, headache, drying of scalp and other *vāyu* diseases. It strengthens the head, forehead, eyes, ears and other sensory organs. The quality of hair improves as they become stronger and smoother and the glow on the face increases. Sesame oil also improves quality of sleep. Combing hair after oiling cleans and beautifies hair[305].

♦ Oil Massage for the body

Just as oiling pots, dry leather and axles of vehicles lubricates and strengthens them, oiling the body makes it stronger and smoothens the skin. The body is protected against diseases caused by *vāyu*. Skin is an organ where *vāyu* accumulates. The pores in the skin that are filled with the heat of *piṭta* absorb the oil applied and calm the *vāyu*. Oiling also destroys premature ageing, fatigue, wrinkles, roughness and dryness. It clears vision, strengthens body, and smoothes skin making it soft and attractive. Oiling also provides relief from body odour, dirt, itching, sweat odour, heaviness and fatigue[306].

Strokes during the massage should be in the direction of the hair growth on the skin. There is no need to apply too much force while massaging. Soft, smooth strokes are adequate. Oiling in the sun speeds up absorption.

---

305. Rathāakṣacharmaghaṭvaḍ bhavanṭyaḅhyaṇgtō guṇaaḥ
Ṣparśanē5ḅhyadhikō vāayuḥ ṣparśanaṃ ça ṭwagāaṣrayaṃ
Ṭvaçhyaṣ́wa paramaḅhyaṇgō yaṣmāaṭ taṃ śēelayēdataḥ
Śiraḥ ṣravaṃa pāadēṣu taṃ viśeēṇa śēelayēṭ
Sa kēśyaḥ śēelitō mōoṛdhani kapāalēṇḍriyatarpaṇaḥ (S. S. Sū 3/57-58)

Ṣhēhāaḅhyaṇgāḍyathāa kuṃbhaśçhçharma ṣnēhavimaṛdanāaṭ
Bhavaṭyupāaṇgāaḍkśaśçha ḍriḍa klēśasahō yathāa
Tathāa śarēramaḅhyaṇgāaḍḍruḍaṃ saṭwaḳ ça jāatyatē
Ṗraśāanṭamāarutāabāadhaṃ ḳlēśavyāayāamasanṣahaṃ (Ch.Su. 5/85-86)

Aḅhyaṇgō maṛsavakaraḥ kaphavāatanirōdhanaḥ
Dhāatōonāaṃ puśṭijananō ṃrijāavaṛṇabalaṗradaḥ (Su. Chi 24/30)

♦ Putting oil in the ears (*karnapurna*)

Ears should be oiled daily. It prevents ailments like deafness, defective hearing, torticolitis, *hanusthambh* and other ear problems. In a healthy ear, oil should be retained for five minutes. When suffering from earache, oil should be retained in the ear till the pain is relieved. This can be done by pressing at the base of the ear to prevent oil from flowing out[307].

♦ Oil Massage of the feet

Oiling feet everyday is very beneficial. It cures roughness, drying, fatigue, lethargy, chapping, shrinking of blood vessels and muscles, sciatica, and other *vāyu* ailments. It also improves eyesight. Its beneficial effects lead the ancient pandits to make it a religious ritual to be performed daily after morning ablutions and before bathing[308].

♦ Putting oil in the nose (*Naṣyakṛiya*)

Nose is considered the entrance to the head. All medicinal preparations pored into the nostrils can reach every nook and cranny of the head. Normally, oil drops should be put in the nostrils in the rainy, winter and spring seasons when there is no cloud cover[309].

---

306. Niṭyaṃ ṣnehārḍara śirasaḥ siraḥśōoklaṃ na jāayatē
Na khāaliṭyaṃ na pāaliṭyaṃ na kēśāaḥ ṗrapataṇti cha
Balaṃ śiraḥ kapāalāanāaṃ viśēēṇābhivardhatē
Ḍriḍmōolāaṣċha D dēeṛghāaṣċha ḳriṣṇāaḥ kāeśāaḥ bhavaṇti cha
Iṇḍriyāaṇi ṗrasēedaṇti suṭwagbhanati chāananaṃ
Niḍrāalāabhaḥ sukhaṃ ċha ṣyāaṇmōorḍhani tāilanisēċvaṇāaṭ *(Ch. Sū 5/81-85)*
Kēśaprasāadhuinēe kēṣyāa rajōjaṇtumalāapahā *(Ṣwaṣthavṛitha saṃnuċhċhaya)*
śirōgtāaṇṣtathāa rōgāaṇċhhirōḅyaṇgō5pakarṣati
Kēśanāaṃ māardavaṃ dāirghyāaṃ bahuṭwaṃ ṣnigdhakriśnatāaṃ
Karoti śarasaṣṭripti ṣuṭwakkamapi chaananaṃ
Saṇterpaṇaṃ chēṇḍriyāṇāaṃ śrasaḥratipōoraṇaṃ *(Su. Chi 24/25-26)*

307. Ṇa karṇarōgāa vāatōṭthāa na manyaahanusangrahaḥ
Noċhċhāiḥ ṣrutirna bāadhiryaṃ ṣyāṇniṭyaṃ karṇapōoraṇaṃ *(Su. Chi 24/29)*

308. ḳharaṭwaṃ ṣtaḅdharāa rāukṣyaṃ ṣramaḥ suptiṣċhapāadayōḥ
Saḍya aivōpaśāaṃyaṇti pāadāḅhayaṇganiṣēvaṇāṭ
jāayatē sāaukumāaryyaṃ ċha balaṃ ṣthāiryaṃ ċha pāadayoḥ
Ḍriṣṭi ṗrasāadaṃ labhate māaarutuśċhōpaśāaṃyati
Na ċha ṣyāadgridṇra5ĕevāataḥ pāadayōḥ ṣphuṭaṇaṃ na cha
Na sirāaṣṇāyusaṇkaṭchaḥ pāadāḅhyaṃgēṇ pāadaayoḥ *(Ch,Su. 5/90-91)*
Niḍrakarō dēchasukhaśċhakṣuśyaḥ ṣramasuptinuṭ
Pāadāaṭwaṇ ṃridukāari ċha pāadāaḅhyaṇgaḥ sadāa hitaḥ *(Su. Chi 24/70)*

309. Varṣē varṣē5n abhaṣṭutēṇutailaṃ ċha kāalēṣu ṭriṣu nāa charēṭ
Ṛrāavṛiṭśaradōo vasaṇtēṣu gatamēghē *(Ch. Sū 6/56)*

This should be done daily after clearing of bowels, cleaning of teeth and oiling of hair. The head should hang back on a chair, and a few drops of warm oil should be put in each nostril using a dropper and inhaled. While pouring get into one nostril, close the other one. Any secretions during *naṣya* should be spat out. After *naṣya*, one must lie on the back till the count of 100 without falling asleep[310]. *Naṣya* cures all ailments that are caused above the neck. Olive oil should be used. Almond oil and *ghēe* made from cow's milk can also be used though they are not as effective. Illnesses like tortocolitis, paralysis, headache, migraine, swelling of the nose, shivering of the head, lock-jaw, etc. are cured. Signs of ageing are not seen and felt in the head and other organs, and greying of hair is prevented[311].

---

310. *Dēṣē vāatarajōmuḳtē ḳritadaṇtanigharṣaṇaṃ*
Viśuḍhaṃ dhōoṇapāanēna swiṇṇamāalagalaṃ tathāa
Uṭtāṇa śāayinaṃ kiṇçhiṭ pralaṃbaśirasaṃ naraṃ
āaṣteěrṇahaṣta pādaṃ ṣcha vasṭrāaçhhāaditalōchanaṃ
Samuṇnamitanāasāa5graṃ vaiḍyā maṣyēṇ yojayēṭ
kāṣṇamaçhhiṇnaḍhāaraṃ ça hēmatāraāḍisuḳtiḅhiḥ
śuḳtyāa vāa yaṭra yuḳtyāa vāa ṗlotāiṛnāa naṣyāaçhaēeṭt
Nasyāṣṇāasiçhayamānēṣu sirō̃ naiva ṗrakaṃpayēṭ
Na kupyēṇna ṗrabhaṣeṭ nōçḥhidēṇna haseṭ tathāa *(Shaa. u. kha 8/47-51)*
Paṇçhaçha sapta daśāiva ṣyaṛmāṭrāa nasyasyaḍhāraṇē
Upaviśyātha niṣṭhōveṇṇāa sā vaḳrra gataṃ ḍravaṃ
Vāamadaḳṣinapāarṣvāḅhyaṃ niṣṭhēevēṭ saṃmukhē na hi
Naṣyē nēetē manaṣṭāpaṃ rajaḥ ḳrodhaṃ ça saṇtyajēṭ
Śayěeṭ niḍrāṃ ṭyaḳṭwāa ça ṗrōṭṭānō nāḳśata naraḥ *(Shaa. U. Kha 8/54-56)*

311. *Na taaṣya çhaḳṣuṛna ghrāṇaṃ ṣrōṭeamupahaṇyatē*
Na syuhṣwētāa na kapilāaḥh kēśaaḥ śam ṣrōoṇi vāa punaḥ
Na cha kēśaaḥ ṗraṃuçhyaṇte vaṛdhaṇtē çha viśeṣataḥ
Naṇyāaṣṭaṃbhaḥ śiraḥ śōolamaṛditaṃ hanusaṇgrahaḥ
Pēehasāaṛdhāavabhēdāu çha śiraḥ kaṃpaṣçha śāaṇyati
Sirāaḥ śiraḥ kapāatāanāaṃ saṇdhayaḥ ṣnāayakaṇdarāaḥ
Nāavanaṗrēeṇitāṣçhāṣya laphaṇte5pyadhikaṃ balaṃ
Mukhaṃ ṗrasaṇṇōpachitaṃ ṣwaraḥ ṣnigdhaḥ ṣtnirō mahāaṇ
Saṛvēṇḍriāaṇaam vāimalyaṇ balaṇ bhavati çhadhikaṃ
Na çhāaṣya rōgāaḥ sahasā ṗrabhanaṇṭyōoṛdhvajatrujaḥ
Jēeṛyataṣṇōṭtamāaṇgēṣu jarāa na labhatē balaṃ *(Ch, Su. 3/28-63)*
Ghanōṇnataṗrasaṇnaṭwaḳṣksṇdhagrěevāasyanaḳṣsaḥ
Sugaṇdhivadanāaḥ ṣnigdhaniṇṣwanāa vimalēṇḍruyāaḥ
Niṛmalēepalitavyaṇgā bhavēyuṛnaṣya śēelinaḥ *(A.S.Su. 3/28-29)*

312. *Kaphapiṭṭāaniladhwaṇsē ṗoorvamaḍhyāa pārāḥṇkē*
Pinē tu grihayatē naṣyaṃ rāaṭrāavaṗyuṭkaṭē gadē *(Sha. u. 8/3)*

Suggested Timings for *Naṣya* Therapy

Kapha aggravation	Dawn	*Piṭta* aggravation	Afternoon
Vāyu aggravation	Night	Autumn and Spring	Dawn
Winter	Afternoon	Summer	Evening
Rainy season	In the sun		

People suffering from *vāyu* ailments that affect the *shiro* like hiccups, *aptāanak*, *maṇyaṣtaṃbh* and hoarseness, should perform *naṣya* twice a day[312].

♦ Exercise

Deliberate physical activity leading to tiring of the body is called Exercise. Exercise lends strength and stability to the body[313]. It should be done daily, in all seasons and according to one's physical capacity. During the winter and spring seasons, it should be done with half the body strength. During summers, rains and autumn, the force applied should be further reduced because these are the seasons of *vāyu* aggravation[314]. To relieve tiredness, the body should be massaged very lightly after exercising. If done keeping the above in mind, exercising is very beneficial. It tones and strengthens every muscle and reduces fat accumulation[315]. Exercising following oil massage aids in absorption. The sweating caused lightens and energises the body. The capacity to work and bear pain increases, digestion is strengthened and body becomes more stable. Aggravated and corrupt *doshas*, especially *kapha*, are calmed[316]. Exercising more than the body strength causes thirst, asthma, cough, fever, bleeding, *klum* (inability of sense organs to function), *shram* (inability of physical organs to function) and vomiting[317]. Excess exercise destroys the body[318], just like a tiger pulling an elephant gets killed.

---

313. śarēerāayāa sujananaṃ karṛ ma vyāaṃa uçhyatē
śarēeraçhēṣṭāa yāa çhēṣṭāa shāiṛyāarthāa balavaṛdhinēe
Dēha vgāyāamasaṇķhyātāa māṭrayāa taaṃ samāahaṛaṭ (ch su 7/31)

314. Aṛḍnśakṭyāa niṣēvyaṣtu balibhiḥ ṣnigdhabhōibhiḥ
śēetakālē vasaṇtē çha maṇdannēva tatās5ṇyadā (A.S.Su. 3/64)
Ṛrāakṣ̣ramāḍ vyāayāmavarjēeṃ cha ṣyāṭ (Ch. Su. 8/18)

315. Lāaghavaṃ kaṛsāaṃṛthyaṃ dēepṭōsgniṛmēdasaḥ ķśayaḥ
Vibhaķtaghanagāaṭraṭnaṃ vyāayāmadupajāyatē (A.S.Su. 62/63)

316. Ṣwēdāagamaḥ ṣ́wāasavṛidhiṛgāaṭraṇāaṃ laghavaṃ tathaa
Hṛidyāaḍyuprōdhaśçha iti vyāyāma lakṣaṇaṃ (Ch. su. 7/33(1)
Uṭsāadanāaṭbhavēṭṣrēehāaṃ viśeṣāaṭkāantimaḍvāampuḥ (Sū chi 24/51-53)
Uḍḍharṣaṇa tu uijgyēyaṃ kaṇḍōokōthāanilāapahaṃ
Ūṛvōḥ sanjanyatyāaśu fēnakaḥ ṣthāiṛlāaghavē

♦ People who should avoid exercise

Vāat-pițta patients, children under 16, adults over 70, and people suffering from starvation. It should also be avoided by people who have lost weight due to walking too much, lifting weights, or excessive sexual activity,[319] Also people under the strain of anger, sorrow, fear and fatigue. Because *Vāyu* and *Pițta* increase during exercise, the above mentioned conditions where *Vāyu* and *Pițta* are already aggravated are unsuitable for exercising. Children are naturally very energetic. So intense exercises like wrestling are to be avoided by them.

♦ Body Pastes

Massaging body with medicated powders and pastes is called *Ubtan*. It is helpful if done before bathing. It destroys *klum*, lends stability to organs by clearing body pores, and smoothes the skin[320]. *Ubtaņ* can be prepared with mustard powder, gram flour, milk, oil, or, curd cream with oil.

♦ Face Packs

Face packs should be applied before bathing to prevent wrinkles, freckles, blackheads and increase softness, glow, uniformity of complexion and shine. It also improves eyesight. Ideally, only a cold face pack should be used. Only during *Vāyu* and *Kapha* aggravation a warm pack should be applied. The pack should be removed when still wet. If it dries, it should be moistened before removal. Removing a dry pack destroys the shine. Sleeping, talking, sitting in the sun or near the fire, getting angry and worrying during face pack application should be avoided because these lead to wrinkle formation. It should also be avoided during indigestion, lock jaw, sinus, indifference, during *nasya* and at night.

Face packs recommended during the six different seasons are:

---

317. *Şramaḥ ķlamaḥ kśgyaştriśņā raķtapițtaṃ prataamakaḥ*
Ativyāyāayaamataḥ kāasōjwarasçhhŗdişçhajāyatē (Ch,Su. 7/33)

318. *Vyāyāamahāşya bhāśyāaḍhuagrāamyadharmaprajāgarāņ*
Nōchitāanapi sēvața budhimāanatimāatŗayāa
Aitāanēuamuidhāanşçhāanyāņ yō5timāaWraṃ nişēnatē
Gajaṃ siṃha ivāakarşaņ sahasā sa vinaśyati (Ch. Su. 7/34-35)

319. *Vāatapițtāamayēe bāalōvŗidhō5jēerņēe çha țtaṃ tyajēț* (A.Su. 3/63)

320. *Dāurganḍhyaņ gāanravaṃ tanḍrāa kanḍōomala marōchakaṃ*
Swēda vēebhatşāaṃ hanti śarēeraparimāarjanaṃ (Ch.Su. 5/93)
Uḍnarrtanaṃ vāataharaṃ kaphamēdōvilāapanaṃ
Sthirēekaraņamangāanaaṃ țwakprasāadakraṃ paraṃ
Sirāamukhavivuiķtatwaṃ țwekşthasyāagnēşçha tējanaṃ
Uḍharşaņōtsāadanāabhayāaṃ jāaayēyāa tāamasanşayaṃ (Su. Sri 24/54-55)

Seasons	Pack
Hemaṇt	Plum seed, adoos *(Adhatoda zeylanica)*, tallow mustard
Shishir	root of *kateri* (*solanum jaquini*), black sesame, turmeric.
Spring	root of *kuśha grass*, sandal-wood, Khus-Khus *(khuś)*, *Albizzia lebbek (shiris)*, anise, *Kaval ki kaṇiyā*
Summer	Red Water Lily *(Kumud)*, *kalhāar*, Conch grass *(dōob)*, Sandal-wood
Rains	*Kaliyak, Sesame, Khus, jata mansi,*
Winter	Indian Valerian *(Tagar)*, *Aquilaria agallocha (Agru)* , *Talees, pundrik,* Liquorice root *(Mulaithi)*

♦ Bathing[321]

Bathing daily is essential for cleaning and refreshing the body. It rejuvenates the body. The nose, ears and feet should be specifically cleaned during bathing. The heat of the koop is absorbed by the body boosting digestive powers and happiness. Thus, bathing helps prolong life. It makes the body mind enthusiastic and increases strength.It prevents fatigue, itching, body odour, sweating, indolence, thirst and irritation[322].

Bathing should be avoided immediately after eating and when suffering from illnesses of eye, mouth and ear, diarrhoea, chronic cold, indigestion, bloating. Bathing aggravates these conditions[323].

---

321. *Paviṭram ṿriśyamāayuśyaṃ śramṣwēdamalāapahaṃ*
śarēerabalasaṇdhāanam snāanamōjaṣkaraṃ paraṃ *(Ch. Sū 5/94)*

Niḍrāa dāahaśramaharaṃ swēdakaṇḍōoṭriṣāapahaṃ
Hridyaṃ malaharaṃ śṛēṣthasṃ saṛvēṇḍriyavibōdhanaṃ
Tanḍrāapāapmōda śamanaṃ tuśṭidaṃ punṣṭwavaṛdhanaṃ
Raḳtaprasāadanaṃ çhāapi ṣhāanamagnēṣçha dēepanaṃ *(Su. Chi 24/57-58)*
Naḍēesu dēvakhāatēṣu tadāagēṣu saraṣṣu ça
Ṣnāanaṃ samāçcharēṇnityaṃ gati pṛaṣravaṇēṣu ça *(Manuḥ)*

322. *Uśṃāaṃbunāa5ḍhaṇkāayaṣya pariṣēkō balāanahaḥ*
Tēnāiva tōoṭtamāangaṣya balahṛita kēśaçhaḳśuṣāaṃ *(As. Su. 3/69-70)*

Uśnēna śirasaḥ ṣnāanaṃhitaṃ çhakśuṣaḥ sadāa
śēetēna śirasaḥ snāanaṃ chakṣuśyamiti niṛdiśēṭ *(Su. Chi 24/59)*

Aśiraṣkaṃ taduṣnēṇ balayaṃ vāatakaphāapahaṃ *(Yogaraṭnākar)*

323. *Snānamaṛdita nēṭrāaṣyakaṛṇarōgāatisāariṣu*
Āadhmānapēenasāajēeṛṇabhuḳta vaṭsu ça gaṛhitaṃ *(A.S.Su.3/75)*
Taçhchatisāara jawaritakaṛṇaśōolāanilāaṛtiṣu
Āaḍhmāanāarōçhakāajēeṛna bhuḳtavaṭsu ça gaṛhitaṃ *(Su. Chi 24/62)*

♦ Clothing

Clean clothes must be worn after bathing. Good, clean and appropriate clothes not only adorn the body, but also bring joy, improve personality and make one fit to appear in gatherings. They also protect the body from the harshness of the seasons. Hence, it is wise to wear clothes according to the seasons. White or light coloured thin clothes in summer and dark, heavy and thick clothes (woollens) in winter[324].

♦ Perfumes & Natural scents

The body can be adorned with seasonal flowers and perfumes. Apart from adding fragrance and attractiveness to the body, they also lift the spirits and increase desire to work. All this ultimately improves the quality of life and longeirty[325].

♦ Wearing Ornaments and Gemstones

As with perfumes, wearing ornaments made of gold, silver, etc. add to the beauty and attractiveness leading to happiness, glow on the face, *mangal* (auspiciousness) and increased life span.

Gemstones like diamonds, *markat*, *goṃed*, etc. should be used. These resolve fear and adverse effect of star/planetatry positions[326].

♦ Chewing Fragranced Substances

To keep mouth fresh and fragranced, substances like nutmeg, betel nut, cardamom, clove, betel leaves, and essence of camphor should be chewed. This also increases taste perception and provides protection against oral diseases[327].

---

324. *Kāaṃyaṃ yaśasyāanāayauśyamalakṣ̣mēeghnaṃ praharṣaṇaṃ*
śrēematpāariṣadaṃ śaṣtaṃ niṛmalaaṃbaradhāaraṇaṃ (Ch. Su. 5/95)
Kadāa5pi na janaḥ sḍdhidhāaryaṃ malinamaṃbaraṃ
Taṭtu kaṇdōokṛimikaraṃ glāaṇyalakṣ̣mikaraṃ paraṃ (Bha Pra Po. 5/931)
Vāaso na dhāarayējēeṛnaṃ malaniṇa raktamulvaṇaṃ
Naāiva ḉhāaṇyēṇ viḍhritaṃ vaṣtraṃ puśpamupāanahāu (A.S.Su.3/34-35)

325. *Vriśyaṃ sāugaṇḍhyamāyuśyaṃ kāaṃjaṃ puśṭibalapradaṃ*
Sāumanaṣyamalakṣ̣mēeghnaṃ gaṇdhamāalyaniṣēvaṇaṃ (Ch. Su. 5/96)
Gaṇdhamāalayāadikaṃ vriśyamalakṣ̣mēeghnaṃ prasāadanaṃ (A.S. Su. 3/34)

326. *Dhaṇyaṃ maṇgalyaṃaayuśyaṃ śrēemaḍvyasanasōodanaṃ*
Harṣaṇaṃ kāaṃuyamōjaṣyaṃ raṭnāabharaṇaḍhāaraṇaṃ (Ch.Su. 5/97)
Raṣē rasāayanē dāanē dhaāraṇē dēvatāaṛchanē
Sulakṣ̣māaṇi sujāatāni savaṛṇāaṇyukṭani śodhayēṭ

327. *Dhāṛyāaṇyāaṣyēna vāiśaḍyaruchi sāugaṇḍhyamiḉhhatāa*
Jāalēekaṭuka pōogāanāaṇ lavaṇgaṣya phalāni cha
Kakkōlaṣya phalaṃ paṭraṃ tāaṃbōolaṣya śubhaṃ tathaa
Tathāa kaṛpōoraniṛyāasaḥ5ōokṣ̣māilāayāaḥ phalāani ḉha (Ch. Su. 5/76-77)
Ruchināiśaḍyasāugaṇḍhyamiḉhhaṇ vakṭrēṇa dhāarayēt
Jaatēe lavaṇgakaṛpōorkaṇkōlakaṭukāiḥ sahaḥ
Tāaṃbōoleenaaṃ kisalayaṃ ḥriḍyaṃ pōogaphalāaṇvitaṃ (A/S/Su. 3/36-37)

♦ Footwear

Footwear protects against heat, cold, thorns, insects and germs, and provides comfort to the feet. They also protect the skin and keep it healthy, and aid in maintaining motion. Footwear should always be comfortable and of the appropriate size[328]. High heeled footwear are not only uncomfortable, they also cause severe disorders. Footwear should be selected according to the season. Appropriate footwear strengthens feet, and makes movement swift and easy.

♦ Nail and Hair Care

Trimming of hair and nails should be a regular habit. Nails are often accumulation points for dirt, germs and toxins. Hence they should be kept as short as possible. This ensures hygiene, beauty and freshness[329].

♦ *Kohl* Application

Eyes should be nourished regularly with kohl or eye drops. Being under constant attack from *kapha dosha* (due to the predominance of the fire element), the eyes benefit from regular application of *kapha*-opposing *kohls* and ointments. Therefore, once every 5-8 days such extract *(rasot)*, should be applied. It makes the eyes water, cleaning them in the process. [Ingredients and procedure for *rasāanjan* preparation[330] – boil and thicken goat milk and turmeric, in the ratio 4:1, cook till it becomes a paste]. This paste also helps relieve eye pain[331]. It should be mixed with honey or water and only a few drops should be used at a time.

It stimulates the eyes and causes tearing.

A few precautions should be taken while

---

328. *Pāadarōgaharaṃ vṛiśyaṃ rakṣ̣ōghnaṃ p̣rēetivaṛdhanaṃ*
Sakhap̣rachāaramōuyaṣyaṃ sadaa pāadatṛadhāaraṇam
Anāarōgyamanāayuśyaṃ chakṣ̣uṣōrōopaghāatakrit̤
Pāadāabhayāamanupāanāaḍbhyāaṃ sadāa ç̣hankramaṇaṇ ṇriṇāaṃ (Su.Ch. 24/71-72)
Pāadukāadhāaraṇaṃ kuṛyāatpōoṛva bhōjanantaḥ param
Pāadarōoharaṃ vṛiśyaṃ ç̣hakṣ̣uśyaṃ chāayuṣ̃hitaṃ
Chakṣ̣uśyaṃ spaṛśanahitaṃ pāadayōṛvyaṣanāapahaṃ
Baḷyaṃ p̣rakṛam sukhaṃ vriśyaṃ pāadaṭradhāaraṇam (Ch. Su. 5/100)

329. *Ṭripakṣ̣asya kēśaṣ̣maṣ̣runakharōmaṇi vaṛdhayēṭ̃*
Na ṣwahaṣṭāina daṇṭāiṛvāa ṣnāanaṃ ç̣hāanusabhaṃarēṭ (A.S.Su. 3/55)
Pāapmōpaśamanaṃ kēśanakharōgamāapamāaṛjanaṃ
Haṛṣalāaghavasāubhāagyakaramuṭsāahavaṛdhanaṃ (Su. Chi 24/73)
Pāu ṣtkaṃ vṛiśyamāayuṣ̃ yaṃ śuchirupavirāajanaṃ
Keśaṣmaṣ̣runakhadēenāaṃ kalpanaṃ saṃprasāadḥanaṃ (Ch. sU. 5/99)

330. *Ç̣hakṣ̣uṣṭējōmayaṃ taṣya viśeṣāaç̣hhalēṣmatō bhayaṃ*
Yojayēṭ saptarāatrē5ṣmāaṭ ṣrāavaṇaartham rasāanjanaṃ (A.S.Su. 3/26)

331. *Sāuvēerāanjanaṃ niṭyaṃ hitanaakṣ̣ṇōoḥ p̣rayōjayēt*
p̣aṇchrāatrēṣṭarāatrē vāa ṣrāavaṇāarthē rasāanjanaṃ (Ch. Su. 5/15)

using kohl. Strong *kohls* should be used only at night as *kapha* formation at this time is low. During the day, excessive watering due to *kohl* application exposes the eyes to the harmful effects of the sun and weakens them[332]. The best time to apply kohl, is dawn as it keeps the eyes soft during the entire day. Kohl made from soot of mustard oil burnt in earthen lamp lends lustre to the eyes, darkens and thickens eyelashes and protects eyes from germs.

♦ Diet

Diet is crucial for maintaining health. Food should always be taken in adequate quantities at the appropriate time, and it should be favourable to one's body constitution. The quantity of food should be guided by one's individual digestive strength and ability.

Some things like green gram are easily digestible. Elements of air and fire are predominant in these 'light' foods. These not only improve appetite, but are also easily assimilated. Hence, eating these substances in large quantities doesn't really cause much harm. But excessive eating does harm digestion. In contrast several food substances like the pulse *uḍad*, etc. are heavy and require time to be completely digested. They are dominated by water and earth elements. They also reduce hunger. Even a slight overeating of heavy foods throws the digestive process out of gear. Though a person with very strong digestion can easily absorb and assimilate heavy foods, it is advised that they be consumed only as much as is sufficient to fill half or three quarters of the stomach. This way, the chance of their causing harm is eliminated[333]. One must eat only after the

---

332. *Divāatṇna prayōḳtavyaṃ netrayōṣteekṣ̣namanjanaṃ*
Virēkaduṛbalāadṛiṣṭirāadityaṃ p̣rāapya sēedari
Taṣmāaṭ ṣrāavyaṃ niśāayāṃ tu dhṛuvamanjanamiśyate (Ch. Su. 5/17)
Ḅhuḳtavāaṇçhhirasāa ṣnāatah̤ śṛāaṇtaṣçhhaṛdanavāahanāiḥ
Rāatrau jaagaritāaṣçhāapi nāaṇjyāajjwarita aiva ç̣ha (Su. Ch. 24/20)
Aṇjana tāabhaḥ :-
Mukhaṇ laghu nirēekṣ̣ēta ḍriḍam paśyati chaḳuṣāa
mataṃ ṣrotō5njanaṃ ṣṛēṣthaṃ vi ṣiudhaṃ sindhusaṃbhavaṃ
Dāahakandōomalaghnaṃ ç̣ha ḍriṣṭiḳtlēdarōojāapahaṃ
Tejōrōopavahaṃ chāiva sahatē māarutāatapāu (Su.Sh. 24/17-18)
Māaṭrāaśēe syāat āahāaramāatrāa punaragnibalāapēkṣ̣iṇēe (Ch. Su. 5/3)
Māaṭrāavaḍḍhāyaśanama śitamanuphaṭya p̣rakritiṃ
balavaṛṇa sukhāayuṣ̣āa yōjayaṭyupayōḳtāaramavaśyamiti (Ch. Su. 5/8)

333. *Na ç̣haivamuḳtē ḍravyē gurulāaghavamakāaraṇaṃ maṇyēta*
laghōoni hi ḍravyāaṇi vāayvagniguṇabahulāani bhavaṇti
P̣rithvēe sōmguṇa bahulāanēetarāani, taṣmāat ṣwaguṇāadapi
Laghōoṇyagnisaṇdhuḳṣ̣naṣwabhāavāaṇyalpadōśāaṇō
Chōç̣hyaṇtē5pi sāuhityōpayuḳtāni, guruṇi panaṛnāagnisaṇdhu
ḳṣ̣naswabhāavāaṇyasāamāaṇyāaṭ ata ṣ̣chāatimāaṭraṃ
dōśakaṇti sāuhityōyayuḳtāaṇyaṇyatra vyāayāamagnibalāatah̤
Sāiṣ̣āa bhavaṭyagnibalaapēkṣ̣eṇēe māatrāa (Ch. Su 5/6)

previous meal has been digested. If these points are kept in mind, food builds and supports the body, improves complexion and general appearance, and increases life span[334]. It also keeps all the *doshas* and *dhātus* in balance leading to a body that is stable and in harmony[335].

♦ Smoking

Ayurved recommends smoking for the following ailments:

Heaviness in the head, headache, swelling of nose, migraine, pain in eyes and ears, hiccups, asthma, night word throat, weak and painful teeth, watering of ear, nose and eyes, smell in nose and mouth, loss of appetite, lock-jaw, torticolitis, itching, infections, pale complexion, premature graying and shedding of hair, baldness, excessive sneezing, too much sleep and laziness, dizziness, heavy voice, etc[336].

In *Ayurved* various preparation prepazations using herbs and medicinal plants to prepare medicated cigars have been described. Drugs and tobacco are not used in their preparation. Such medicated smoking provides nourishment to hair, skull, voice and strengthens sense organs. It also protects against throat and head ailments caused by *Vāyu* and *Kapha doshas*[337].

---

334. *Na cha nāapēkṣtē ḍravyaṃ ḍravyāapēkṣayāa cha tribhāaga*
Sāuhiṭyamardhasāuhiṭyaṃ vāa guruṇāmupadiśyatē **(Ch. Sū 5/7)**

335. *Kāalaṣtu ṛituvyāaḍhyapēkṣō jēerṇāajēerṇa lakṣaṇaśçha* **(A S.Su 10/11)**
Ajēerṇaṃ hi pōoṛvaṣyāahāaraṣyāaparinṭō rasa uṭtaṛeṇa
Saṃṣrijyamāanaḥ
Ṣaṛvāaṇ dōśaaṇ prakōpayaṭyāaśu **(A. S.Sū 10/12)**

336. *Gāurav śirasaḥ śōolaṃ pēenasāaṛdhāavabhāidakāu*
Kaṛnāakśiśōolaṃ kāasaśçha hiḳkāaśwāasāu galagrahaḥ
Daṇtadāuṛbalayamāaṣrāavaḥśrōṭraghṛaṇāakṣidōśajaḥ
Pōotiṛghrāaṇāaṣyagaṇḍhaśçha daṇta śōolamarōchakaḥ
Hanumaṇyāagrahaḥ kaṇdōoḥ ḳrimayaḥ pāaṇdutāa mukhē
Ślēṣma praśēkō vāiṣvaṛya galaśvṇḍyupajihikāa Khāaliṭyaṃ piṇjaraṭwaṃ
çhakēsāanāaṃ pataṇaṇtathaa
Śravathōoṣçhāatitaṇḍrāa ça buḍḍhēṛmōhō5tiniḍratāa
Dhōomapāanāatāpraśaāṃyaṇti balaṃ bhavati chāadhikaṃ
Śirōrōohakapāalāanāamiṇḍriyāaṇaaṃ ṣwarasaṣya çha
Na çha vāata kaphāaṭmanō balinō5pyōoṛdhvajatrujāa
Dhōomavaḳtra kapāanaṣya vyāaḍhyaḥ ṣyuḥ Śirōgatāaḥ **(Ch. Sū 5/27-32**

337. *Navanāaṇjananiḍṛāaṇṭē çhāaṭmavāaṇ dhōomapō bhavēṭ*
Tathāa vāatakaphāaṭmāanō bhavaṇtyōoṛdhvajatrujaaḥ **(Ch. Sū 5/35)**
Ṛrayōgikaṃ tato dhōomaṃ gaṇdhamāayāadi chāachrēṭ
Dhōomāadaṣyōṛḍhvajatrāotthāa na ṣyuṛvāatakaphāamayāaḥ **(A. S. Sū 3/32)**

338. *Ṛrayōgapāanē tasyāaśṭāu kāalāaḥ saṃparikēeṛtitaḥ*
Ṣnāaṭwāa bhuḳtwāa saṃmulḷikhya ḳśuṭwāa danṭāaṇnighriśya cha **(Ch. Su. 5/33)**

There are 8 periods during a day suitable for smoking[338]. Smoke can be inhaled after bathing, cleaning of tongue, brushing, eating, sneezing, explain, kohl application and sleeping. Inhaling thrice is recommended at every smoking session[339].

When done properly, the chest, throat and head feel lighter and *kapha* melts and is eliminated[340]. Too much smoking heats and dries the tongue, throat and head. Sense organs become heated and thirst increases. Dizziness, loss of consciousness and bleeding might also be experienced[341]. Therefore, smoking should be done very carefully.

♦ Behaviour : what is good conduct

To remain healthy and happy, one must live a life guided by *dhaṛma*. *Dhaṛma* (being righteous and moral), *aṛth* (acquiring material wealth) and *kāam* (gratifying desires), should be done in a way that is not mutually conflicting. Truth must be practised at all times. Every creature, including things as tiny as ants and insects, must be considered equal and treated with respect. One must always be ready to help the poor, sick and people who have suffered loss. One must never disappoint those who ask for help or insult them. God, cattle, holy man, the old,women, children, doctors, king and guests must always be respected and protected[342].

One must never possess things belonging to others or even desire them[343]. One must guard against sinning and avoid ill-treating even bad individuals. Weaknesses and secrets of others should not be revealed. Company of treacherous, corrupt, wicked, depraved, miserly and evil individuals should be avoided. People who think of the universal welfare should be befriended and approached for advice. On the other hand, one must always be careful of those who have disruptive tendencies[344].

---

339. *Rogāaṣtaṣya tu pēyaah̤ ṣyurāapāanāaṣtriṣṭrayaṣtrayah̤*

340. *Ḥriṭkaṇthēṇḍriya saṇśudhiṛlaghuṭwaṃ śirasah̤ śamah̤*
Yathēritāanāaṃ dōośāaṇaam saṃyakapēetaṣya lak ṣaṇam (Ch. Su 5/37)

341. *Bāadhiryamāaṇḍhyamōokaṭwaṃ rah̤tapiṭtaṃ siroḅhramaṃ*
Akāalē chaatipēetaśçha dhōomah̤ kuṛyāadupaḍravāaṇ (Ch. Su 5/38)

342. *Saṭyavāadinaṃ ķrodhaṃ niṿoritaṃ maḍḍyamāithunāaṭ*
Ahiṇsakamanāayasaṃ p̣raśaaṇtaṃ p̣riyavāadināaṃ

343. *Japaśāuchaparaṃ dhēeraṃ dāananiṭyaṃ tapaṣvinaṃ*
Dēvagōḅrāah̤maṇāachāaṛyaguruṿriḍhāarçhanē rataṃ

344. *Dēsakāalap̣raṃāaṇajgyaṃ yuḳtiggyamanahaṇķritaṃ*
Śaṣṭāachāaramasaṇkēeṛṇamaḍhyāaṭma p̣ravaṇēṇḍriyam
Upāasitāaraaṃ ṿridhāanāamāaṣṭikāanāaṃ jitāaṭmanāaṃ
Dhaṛmaśāaṣtraparaṃ viḍyāaṇnaraṃ niṭyarasāayanaṃ (Ch. Chi 1-4/33-34)

♦ What Conduct Should Be Avoided

❖ Climbing trees and dangerous mountain roads, travelling in dangerous vehicles, bathing in forceful flowing rivers[345].

❖ Sleeping on uncovered, small, uneven and pillowless bed[346].

❖ Stepping over a relative, person of high birth, teacher, guide, holy person, sacred trees, and the shadow of a person is inauspicious[347].

❖ Transgressing by keeping sacred things and people on the left while putting other things on the right.

❖ Laughing loudly in a gathering, burping or passing gas noisily, yawning, coughing or sneezing without covering the mouth, cleaning nostrils, letting teeth chatter, scratching mud, cracking joints, keeping limbs in awkward positions and moving them ungracefully, etc[348].

❖ Staring at shiny objects, planets, undesirable, impure and censured objects[349].

❖ Staying late at night in– temples, sacred places, gardens, crossroads, graveyards and lonely places[350].

❖ Venturing alone in a jungle or slaughter-house.

---

345. *Nagirivişamamaştakēşvanucharēţ, nadrumamāarōhēţ, najalōgravēgamavagāahēţ* *(Ch. Su. 8/19)*
Purōvāatāataparaņştusāarapuruşaanilāaņ
Anujaḥ kşvathudgāarakāasaşwapnāatramāithunaṃ
Saśabdamanilaṃ haştamrōonetrāţkşēpavāaditaṃ
kōolachhāayāaṃ surāapāanaṃ vyāalaṃdaştrivişāaņinaḥ
Haninās̄aryāatinipuņasēvaṃ vigrahamuttamāiḥ
Sandhyāaşwabhyavahāaraştrēeşwapanāadhyayanachiņtanaṃ
Āarōgyajēevitāiśyavarya vidyāasuşthiramāanitāaṃ
Tōyāagnipōojyamodhēna yāana dhōomaṃ vāaśrayaṃ
Maghāatisakti vişrambhaşwāatantrayē ştrēeşu cha tyajēt *(Ch. A. S3/108-111)*

346. *Na jāanusamaṃ kathinamāasanamadhyāasēeţ*
nāanāaştēerņamanupahitamavi sāalasamaṃ vāa śayanaṃ prapadyēţ *(Ch. Su. 8/19)*

347. *Nāaspriştvāaratnāajyamangalasumanasō5bhinişkrāamēţ*
Na pōojyamangalāanyapasavyaṃ gachhēnnetarāanyanudakşiņaṃ *(Ch. Su 8/19)*
Na vriddhāanna gurōonna gaņāannanripāaņ vāa adhikşipēţ *(Ch. Su. 8/25)*

348. *Nōchchāiŗhasēţ na śabdavantaṃ māarutaṃ muchyēţ*
Naa nāavritamukhō jriṃbhāaṃ kşavathu hāasyaṃ vāa pravartayēţ *(Ch. Su. 8/99)*

349. *Satataṃ na nirēekşēţ chala5ookşmāapriyāaņi cha*
Nāapraśaştaṃ na viņmōotraṃ na darpaņamamāarrjitoṃ *(A. S. Sū 3/100)*
Jyotēenşyanişţanmēdhyamaśaştaṃ cha nāabhivēekşēţ *(Ch. Su 8/19)*

350. *Na vyāalāanupasarpēņna danştrinō na vişāaņinaḥ* *(Ch. Su 81/9)*
Na kşapāaşwamarasadanachāityachatwara chatu spathō
Pawan sma saanāadyāatanāanyāasēvēta nāikaḥ śōonyagrahaṃ na chāatavēemanupraviśeţ *(Ch. Su 8/19)*

- Maintain distance from snakes, animals with sharp horns and teeth, and fire. One must stay away from fire when upset and after meals, especially if hands and mouth are unwashed.
- Protect against wind from the East, sun, hail and wind storms.
- Showing strength or courage more than one's potential, bathing and sleeping more than required, staying awake at night, intake of excessive liquids[351].

Other things to be avoided- improper conduct, befriending wicked people, alienating good people, sitting for long with, knees up, keeping fire under bed for heating, bathing without removing all clothing and without cleaning mouth, and wearing the same clothes after a bath[352].

♦ Precautions While Studying

Appropriate time and light should be arranged while studying. Light source should always be on the left or behind. Studying should be avoided at places where something is burning, during earth quake, solar and lunar eclipse, important festivals, dusk and[353] daybreak. Body posture and position of the book is very important. The reading material should be at least a foot away from the body. Reading while lying down weakens the eyesight. Care should be taken to keep the pronounciation clear and complete. Voice should not be too loud or too soft, or too harsh also. Reading should not be done too forcefully or too languidly[354]. Recitation should be neither too fast nor too slow and with necessary intonations.

Norms of Good Conduct

No one should break the universally accepted laws of behaviour.

- Roaming at night and at unseemly places is inappropriate.
- Eating, studying, sleeping and sex at dawn and dusk is prohibited[355].
- Alcohol, gambling and attraction towards prostitutes should be avoided[356].
- Insulting someone, being unfriendly and

351. *Na sāahasāatiṣwapnaprajāagaraṣnāanapāanāanyāasēvēṭ noṛḍhwajāanuṣchiraṃ tiṣṭhēṭ* *(Ch. Su 8/19)*

352. *Niṭyaṃ anuhatavāasāaḥ sumanāaḥ sugaṇḍhiḥ ṣyāat* *(Charak Su. 8/18)*

353. *Na viḍyuṭṣwanāaṛtavēeṣu nāaḅhyuditāasu diḳsu nāagnisamṗlavē na bhōomikaṃpē na mahōṭsavē nōlkāapāate Na mahāagrahōpagamanē na baṣṭacḥaṇḍrāayāaṃ tithāu na sanḍhyayōṛ nāamakhāaḍ gurōṛnāavapatitaṃ* *(Ch. Sa. 8/24)*

354. *Na viṣwaraṃ nāanavaṣthitapāadaṃ nāatiḍrutaṃ na vilaṃbitaṃ nāatiḳlēebaṃ Nāaṭyuchḥāiṛnāatinēecḥāiḥ swarāiraḍhyayanamaḅhyaśyēṭ* *(Ch. S. 8/24)*

355. *Saṇḍhyāaṣwaḅhyavahāaraṣṭrēeṣwapnāaḍhyayana cḥinṭanaṃ* *(A.S. Su. 3/111)*

356. *Na maḍyaḍyōotavēśyāaprasaṇgaruchiḥ ṣyāaṭ, na guhyaṃ viṿriṇuyāata na kaṇchidavajāanēeyāaṭ Nāahaṇmāanēe ṣyāaṇnāadaḳṣō nāadaḳṣiṇā nāasōoyakaḥ* *(Ch. Su 8/25)*

behaving rudely due to excessive pride is wrong.

- ❖ Indulging in slander and using harsh words against old people, teachers, leaders and against anyone in a gathering is uncivilised.
- ❖ Being talkative, impatient and too aggressive is improper.
- ❖ Dependants and subordinates should be taken care of and not looked down upon[357].
- ❖ Blind faith, suspicious nature and being dependent are harmful[358].
- ❖ Careful planning before undertaking a new project is highly recommended. Once a job is undertaken, delaying, postponing and leaving it unfinished should be avoided[359].
- ❖ Dignity should be maintained in both success and defeat.
- ❖ Working with excessive happiness or immense anger must be avoided. Being too sensitive about petty things is not healthy.
- ❖ One must not become a slave to one's senses. However, suppression of desires must also not become a regular habit.
- ❖ One must act according to one's nature and character.
- ❖ Self-respect is good. But one must steer clear of constantly thinking about past insults.
- ❖ One must have abiding faith in the cause and effect theory (good results from good, and bad from evil), and this should become the guiding principle of all actions.
- ❖ Character, behaviour and habits should not be questionable. Private parts must not be exposed[360].
- ❖ One must share one's joys[361] with others.

Who to Befriend?

Friendship should be cultivated with :-

- ❖ Individuals with experience, wisdom, intelligence, pure conduct, patience, strong memory, good concentration.
- ❖ Those who have attained knowledge and maturity or those who have the company of such people.
- ❖ Those who are calm, remain free from worries and stress, and know good behaviour from bad.
- ❖ Those whose behaviour is impeccable and who always work for common welfare.
- ❖ Those that support good conduct and whose name and philosophy is revered.

---

357. *Na chāatibrōoyāaṭ, na bāaṇdhavāanuraḳtakṛiçhhra ḍwitēeyaguḥyajg̦yāana bahiṣ́kuryāaṭ* (Ch. S. 8/25)

358. *Na saṛvaviṣ́ṛaṃbhēe na saṛvāabhiśaṇkēe na saṛvakāalavichāari* (Ch. S 8/26)

359. *Na chāatidēeṛghasōotrēe ṣyāaṭ* (Ch. S. 8/27)

360. *Na guḥyaṃ viṿriṇuyāaṭ* (Ch. S. 8/25)

361. *Niṛbhēekaḥ, ḥvēemāaṇ dhēemāaṇ mahōṭsāahaḥ dakṣ́sah*
Ḳśmāavāaṇ dhāaṛmikaḥ āaṣtikaḥ, uinayabuddhiviḍyāabhijanavayō
-ṿriḍḍha siḍḍhāachāaṛyāamupāasitāa (Charak Su. 8/18)

♦ Persons Not To Be Befriended

Those that lack the qualities enumerated above and who are wicked, interested in bad deeds, use foul language, have unethical thoughts, indulge in criticism and slander, are quarrelsome, greedy, envious, fickle-minded, cruel and unkind[362] should not be friended.

2. *Ratricharya*
(Pattern of behaviour and food habits at night)

12 hours of daylight and 12 hours of darkness are together referred to as one day. Hence *ratricharya* is similar to *dincharya.*

Sleep is described first, since the primary activity at night is sleeping.

♦ Sleep

It is common knowledge that to maintain good health and spirits sound and adequate sleep is crucial. On completing all tasks scheduled for the day, both the mind and the body are fatigued, and both the sense and motor organs are drained[363]. This induces a desire to sleep. Therefore, the state when the mind loses communication with sense and motor organs due to which they become inactive is called *sleep*. During sleep only the most vital processes like breathing, blood circulation, etc. continue to be performed; the rest are suspended. Energy is thus conserved leading to recharging of body strength. This accounts for the high energy levels and the feeling of freshness after a good night's rest.

Night-time is the most conducive for sleep as the *Kapha dosha* in the body and *tamas dosha* in the mind help to induce sleep[364]. The silence, darkness and lower temperatue during night increases the levels of the two *doshas* in the body, leading to sound sleep.

Sleep Types	
Dream state	This is a state when a person dreams and the restless mind remains active engaging in thinking and worrying. This 'type' is not sound sleep and hence not relaxing[365].
in deep sleep *(Sushupt)* state	All activities of the mind and body are in suspension.

---

362. *Na lōkabhōopaviḍviṣṭāiṛna saṇgaçhhēta nāaṣṭikaḥ*
Kali vāiraruchinaṛna ṣyāaḍḍhēerah sampāaḍvipaṭtiṣu **(A. San. Su. 382)**

363. *Yadāa tu manasi kṭaanṭē kaṛmāaṭmāanaḥ kḷamāaṇvitāa*
Viṣayēḅhyō nivaṛtaṇṭē tadāa ṣwapiti māanavaḥ **(Ch. Su. 21/35)**

A *sushupt* state of even a very short duration is extremely refreshing. It reinvigorates both the mind and the body[366]. On the other hand, even a long period of dream state fails to provide rest or refresh the body.

Together with physical fatigue caused by hardwork, mental peace is absolutely essential to enjoy sound sleep. Those who cannot sleep, suffer from insomnia that causes several mental and physical disorders[367].

Insomnia – Causes

- ❖ Mental disturbances like fear, worry, sorrow and anger
- ❖ Excessive physical labour, exercise or fatigue
- ❖ Bloodletting
- ❖ Fasting too much
- ❖ Smoking
- ❖ Uncomfortable bed or resting place
- ❖ Excessive *satva guna* and low *tamo guna*
- ❖ Old age ailments caused by *Vāyu* aggravation like *shōol*, *pēedā* etc.
- ❖ Loss of *doshas* due to loose motions and vomiting
- ❖ Natural tendency towards sleeplessness[368]

---

364. *Ḥriḍayaṃ chētanāa ṣthāanamuḳtaṃ suṣrutāadēhināaṃ*
Tamō5ḅhibhōotē taṣmiṣtu niḍrāaviśati dēhinaṃ
Niḍrāa hētū ṣtamaḥ saṭtvaṃ bodhanē hēturōochyatē
Ṣwabhāava aiva vāa heturgarēeyāaṇ parikēerṭyate (Su. Sha. 4/34)

365. *Pōoṛvadēhāambhōotāaṇṣtu bhōotāaṭmāa ṣwapataḥ ṗrabhuḥ*
Rajoyuḳtēna manasāa grahḷāaṭyaṛthāaṇśubhāa śubhāana
Karaṇāanāaṃ tu vāikalyē tamasāabhi pravaṛdhitē
Aṣwapaṇnapi bhōotāaṭmāa ṗrasupta iva ċhōċhyāṭē (Su. Sha. 4/36)

366. *Dēha viśṛayatē yaṣmāaṭtaṣmāaṇnidāa ṗrakēeṛtitāa*
Niḍrāaṇtu vāiśṇavēe pāapmāanamupadiśaṇti śāa
ṣwabhāata aiva saṛvapraṇinō5bhi ṣpriśati (Su. Sha 1)
Sāiva yuḳtāa panaṛyunḳtē niḍrāa dēhaṃ sukhāayuṣāa
Puruṣaṃ yōginaṃ siḍḍhayāa saṭyāa buḍḍhirivāagatāa (Ch. Su 21/38)
Bhōjanāanaṇtaraṃ niḍrāa vāataṃ harati piṭṭaṇṇaṭ
Kaphaṃ karōti vapuṣaḥ puṣṭiṃsāuḳhyaṃ tanōtihi (Cha. Pra. 5/220)

367. *Niḍrāanāaṣāadaṇgmaṛda śirōgāuravajṛiṃbhikāaḥ*
Jāadyaṃ glāanibḥramāapaḳtinḍrāarōgāaṣċha vāatajāaḥ (Vaa. Su. 7/63-64)
Asāaṭmyāajjāagarāaṛḍhaṃ ṗraataḥ ṣwapyāaḍbhuḳtavāaṇ (Vaa Su. 7/65)

Treatment
❖ Massage, *Ubtan* (medicated pastes) application, and pressing of limbs.
❖ Intake of slightly oily foods, curd and *shāali (a kind of rice)*, rice, milk and alcoholic drinks
❖ Mental peace
❖ Listening to selected music
❖ Applying soothing ointments and pastes over eyes, head and face
❖ Sleeping in a quite and comfortable place
❖ Inhaling perfumes or scents.

♦ Avoid Sleeping During the Day

Sleeping during the day is harmful for health as it increases *kapha* and *piṭta doshas* leading to various illnesses[369] like severe jaundice, headache, heaviness, body-ache, weakening of digestion, congestion in the chest region, swelling, lack of appetite, vomiting, nauseous feeling, swelling of nose, migraine, urticaria *(shēetpiṭta)* or *(ḉhhapāki)*, boils, itching, languor, cough, throat ailments,[370] blunting of

368. *Kāayaṣya śiraṣaṣḉhāiva virēka ṣḉhhaṛdanaṃ bhayaṃ*
Chiṇṭāakṛōdhaṣtathāa dhōomō vyāayāamō raktamōkśaṇaṃ
Upavāasō5sukhāa śayyāa saṭvāudāarya tamōjaḥ
Niḍrāaprasaṇgamahitaṃ vāarayaṇti samuṭthitaṃ
Aita aiva ḉha vijgyēyāa niḍrāanāaśaṣya hētavaḥ
Kāarya kāalō vikāaraṣḉha ṗrakṛiti vāayuṛēva ḉha (Ch. Su. 21)
Virēkaḥ kāayśira sōṛvamaṇaṃ raktamōksāaṇaaṃ
Dhōomkśuṭ riṇṭyathāa haṛṣaśōkāmāithunabhēe kṛuḍḍhaḥ
Chintōṭkaṇthāa5sukhāa śayyāa saṭyāudāarya tamōjayaḥ (A. S. Su. 9/53)
Rōokṣṇnaṃ ḉhāahitāaṃ niḍrāaṃ vāarayaṇti ṗrasanaiganēeṃ (A. S. Su. 9/54)
Kāalaśēela kśyō vyāadhiṛvriḍḍhiṣḉhāanilapitayōḥ (A.S. Su. 9/55)

369. *Akāalē5tiprasaggāaḉhcha na cha niḍrāa niṣēvitāa*
Sukhāayuṣēe parāakuṛyāaṭkāalarāatririvāaparāa (Ch. Su. 21/37)
Divāa ṣwapṇō hitō5ṇyaṣmina kaphapiṭtakarō hi saḥ (A. S. Su. 9/45)
Mukṭamāaṭraṣya ḉha ṣwapṇāaṣḍwaṇṭyagni kupita kapha (Maa. Ni)
Taṣmāaṭrajāagriyāaḍrōoṭrāu dināaṣwapnaṃḉha vaṛjayēṭ
Jgyāaṭwāa dōśakarāavētāu budhaḥ ṣwapṇaṃ mitaṃ charēṭ (Su. Sha 4/38)

370. *Halēemaka śsirahśōolaṇṣtāimitya gurugāaṭratāah* (Ch.S. 21/46)
Jwarabḥramamatibḥraśaṇṣtrōtōrōdhāagnimaṇdatāa
Śōphāarōḉhaka ḥrilḷāasapēenasāaḍhavibhedaka (A.S. Su. 9/50)
Kaṇdōorōokḳōthapiṭtakāa kāasatauḍrāagalamayāaḥ
Viṣavēga ṗravṛiṭṭiṣḉhāa bhavēdahitaniḍrayāa (A.S.Su. 9/51)
Akāalaśayabāaṇmōhajwarṣtāimityapēenasāaḥ (Va. Su. 9)
Śirōrōokṣō hrilḷāasa ṣtrōtōrōdhagnimaṇdatāa (Ch. Su.)

memory and intelligence, blockage of various body channels, fever, weakening of sensory and motor organs, increased vulnerability to toxins etc. People who are overweight, are used to an oily diet, suffer from *kaphaj* ailments on account of having *kapha* dominated *pṛakṛiti*, have arthṛitis or suffer from artificial poisoning, must never sleep during the day[371].

♦ Exceptions

Due to loss of water and shorter nights, sleeping during the day in summers is not harmful. There are some other conditions when sleeping during day time is not prohibited[372] - after rigorous music practice, studying, walking; consumption of alcoholic substances, suffering from weakness, fatigue, thirst, diarrhoea, shooting pains *(shōol)*, asthma, hiccups; weak constitution during childhood and old age, suffering from injury, lack of sleep during night, being drained due to anger, fear or sorrow. Under such conditions, the strength of the body and the *dhātus* remain in balance.The *kapha dosha* nourishes the organs and the lifespan increases[373].

♦ Rules for Eating Dinner

Digestion of food and sleep are inextricably linked[374]. Keeping in mind the fact that indigestion hampers sleep, food should be taken as early as possible. A two-hour gap between dinner and sleep is a must. Only light and easily digestible food should be eaten. Walking after dinner is recommended. It improves digestion and therefore aids sound sleep[375].

♦ Avoid Curd at Night[376]

Despite being beneficial normally, curd has a tendency to block body channels. Hence eating curd at night should be avoided as one has to sleep after dinner. The digestive process continues at a very slow pace during sleep. The chances of *srotas* (body channels) getting blocked increases. Consequently sleep and digestion are disrupted. Even healthy people

---

371. *Bahunēdaḥ kaphāaḥ ṣwapyuḥ ṣnēhaniṭyāaṣçha vāahani*
Viṣāarṭtaḥ kaṇṭharōgēe çha nāiva jāatu niśāaṣwapi *(A.S.Su. 9/48)*

372. *Çrēeṣmē vāayuçhayāadāanarāuķśyarāaṭrayalpabhāavataḥ*
Divāaṣwapnō hitō5ṇyaṣmiṇ kaphapiṭṭakarō hi saḥ *(A. S. Su. 9/45)*

373. *Mōokaṭwāatiyāaśpayāandhwamadhaṣṭrēe bhāarakaṛmbhiḥ*
krodhaśōkabhayāiḥ klāanṭāaṇ swāasahidhmāaśtisāariṇaḥ *(A. Su. 9/46)*
Vriddha bāalāabalakśēeṇa ṣatatriṭçhhlapēeditāan
Ajēerṇya5bhikritōṇmatāana divāaṣwapnōchitāanapi
Dhāatusamaṃyaṃ tayāa hyēṣāa ślēṣmāa çhāaṇgani puśyati *(As. Su. 9/47)*

374. *Ṭraya upaṣṭaṃbhāa iti āahāaraḥ ṣwapnōḥ bṛahmacharyamiti* *(Ch. Su. 11/35)*

375. *Rāaṭrēe tu bhojanaṃ kuṛyāaṭprathamapraharāanṭarē*
Kiçhchidōonaṃ samaṣṇēeyāaḍ duṛjaṛaṃ tatra varjayeṭ *(Bha. Pra.)*
Sāayaṃ bhukṭwāa laghu hitaṃ samāahitamanāaḥ śudhiḥ
Śāaṣṭāaramanusaṇṣṃritya ṣwaśayyāaṃ chāaya saṇviśēṭ *(A.S. Su. 3/120)*

376. *Na nakṭaṃ dadhi bhuṇjēeṭ na chaapyaghrtaśaṛkaraṃ*
Nāamuḍgayuṣaṃ nāakśāuḍraṃ nōṣṇaṃ nāamalakāiṛvināa
Jwarāaṣrikipitta vēesaṛpa kuśṭha pāaṇdu vayabhramāaṇ *(Ch. Su. 7/61)*
Pṛaapnuyāaṭ kāamalāaṃ chōgrāaṃ vidhiṃhiṭwāa dahipriyaḥ *(Ch. Su. 7/62)*

must therefore avoid eating curd at night. Patients of asthma, cough, cold and arthritis must not eat curd even during the day as these disorders are caused due to the blocking of the *srotas*.

♦ Studying At Night:

Adequate light while studying is a must to ensure healthy eyesight. But it must be remembered that sunlight is far better than artificial light,which weakens eye power gradually overtime As far as possible, studying at night should be kept to the minimum[377]. Writing is more stressful on the eyes; hence it should be avoided at night.

Sexual Activity[378]

Ayuṛved places certain limits on sexual activity dictated by health concerns and rules of social conduct. Sexual activity should be avoided under the following circumstances:

- During menstruation or when suffering from infection or disease
- With bad characters, unattractive and others.
- In case of lack of friendly feeling, lack of sexual desire, attraction to another male or married woman or with a woman belonging to another caste
- In sacred places, public areas, crossroads, gardens, graveyards, slaughter houses, water spots, hospitals, temples and residences of *Brāḥman*, teacher and guide.
- At dawn, dusk, full moon nights, nights of the new moon, (first day of the fortnight), and eight day of the lunar cycle *(ashthmi)*
- The male being in impure state or suffering from low libido
- While not consuming milk or some other to cause swelling (vriśya) substance
- Without eating or after overeating
- While fasting, after physical labour or experiencing fatigue or a strong urge to urinate
- In inappropriate places, or lack of privacy[379]

Sexual intercourse with other than sexual organs is prohibited. A glass of milk with sugar or honey should be taken before and after intercourse[380].

---

377. *Na Saṇḍhayayōṛnāamukhāadguṛōṛnāavapatitaṃ* (Ch. Su. 8/24)
Na Saṇḍhyāaṣwaḅhya vahāaṛāaḍhyayanaṣtrēe ṣwapnasēvēe syāaṭ (Ch. Su. 8/25)

378. *Ģrāaṃyadhaṛma pṛavṛitāu tu rajaṣwalāamaniṣṭāaçhāaṛāa*
maśaṣṭāamatiṣthōolāamaḳriśāaṃ gaṛbhiṇēeṃ sōotikāamanuṭṭāanaṃ
Viḳritāaṇgēe gaṇikāamapṛajasaṃ ḍuṣṭayōnimaṇyayōnimaṇyaṣtriyaṃ
Viśeṣāaçhça vayō vaṛṇavṛiḍḍhāaṃ sagōtṛāaṃ (A.S. Su. 9/169)
Rajaṣwalāamakāamāaṇcha malināamapṛiyāaṃ tathāa
Vaṛṇavṛiḍḍhāaṃ Vayōvṛiḍḍhāaṃ tathāa vģāadhipṛapēeḍitāaṃ (Su. Chi 24/114)

3. Ritucharya
(Food and behavior patterns during different seasons)

Seasons and environment affect our health as much as food. The state of *doshas* in the body changes with the seasons. Due to the reduction, aggravation and calming of the *doshas* as a result of seasonal change, *Ayurved* recommends different food and behaviour patterns for different times of the year. Following these rules is crucial to maintain health and to protect oneself from sickness[381].

India experiences three seasons during a year – summer, winter and rains. Changes in human body occur according to the seasons. The three seasons are further divided into six types – spring (*basant*), summer (*grišhm*), rains (*varsha*), autumn (*sharad*), winter (*hemaṇt*) and extreme cold (*shishir*). The seasons are based on the movement of the sun, known as *ayan*[382]. *Ayan* is of two types:

1. ***Uṭtarāyan*** – During *uṭtarāyan*, the sun moves towards the north. This is also called the *āadaan* period as the sunrays and winds are very hot and dry and absorb moisture rapidly. The effects of these conditions are felt by all vegetation and the human body as well. It depletes energy and causes weight loss. This period includes extreme cold , spring and summer[383].

2. ***Dakshināyan*** – During this period the

---

379. *Hēenāangēe garbhiṇēem ḍwēśyāaṃ yōnidōśasamaṇvitāaṃ*
Sagōtrāaṃ gurupaṭnēem ċhatathāa pravrajitāamapi (Su.Chi 24/115)
Tathāa chāiṭyaċhaṭwara chatuśpathōpawana śmaśaanāayaṭana
Salilāuṣadhiḍwijagurusuraṇripāalayēśvahani-gōsargē
maḍhyaṇdinē5ṛḍharāatrē parvadinēṣvanangē, pipāasurapraṇēeta
Saṇkalpō vāa na gaċhhēta (A.S. Su. 9/69)

380. *Ṣnāanāangarāagavyajanēṇdupāadamāasāasavakṣēeran rasāalāaṃ*
Bhakṣmāan sitāadhyāan salilaṃ suśēetaṃ
Sēvēṭ nidrāaṃ ċha ratāantatāantaḥ (A.S. Su 9/76)
Ṣnāanulēpahimāaṇikhaṇda ṣwāahāa śēetaṃbuduṃdharasayōoṣa
Surāaprasannāa sēvēṭ (Aṇya āchāarya)

381. *Taṣyāaśotāadyāadāahāarāadbalaṃ varna ṣċha vardhatē*
Yaṣyartusāaṭmyaṃ viditaṃ ċhēṣṭahāara vyapāaṣrayaṃ (Ch. Su. 6/3)
Charadhāatōgati bhakśaṇāarthaṣya ċharyamiti rōopaṃ
Tēn āahāarō vihāarāa ċharaśaṣdēnēeċhyatē (A.S. Su. 4/Dalhan)

382. *Iha khalu saṃ—vaṭsaraṃ ṣadangamrituvibhāagēṇ viḍyāaṭ*
Taṭrāadiṭyāaṣyōḍgayanamāadāanaṃ ċha ṭrēenṛituṇċhhiśirāadēeṇ
Ġrēeṣmāantāaṭ vyavaṣyēṭ varṣāadēeṇ punarhēmantāantāan
dakṣiṇāayana visargacha (Cu. Su. 6/4)
Ta aitē śēetō ṣṇavarṣāa lakśaṇāaśċhaṇdrāadiṭyōḥ
Kāalavibhāagakaraṭwāadayanē ḍwē bhavatō dak ṣiṇamuṭtaraṃcha (Ch. Su)

sun moves towards the south. Sunrays and winds are neither hot nor dry. The effect of moon is prominent. The temperature decreases and the weather is pleasant and mild. Wind, clouds and rains cool down. This is called the *visarg* period. Due to the cooling down of the environment, food and medicinal preparations acquire a smoothness which results in an increase in physical strength in both animals and humans[384].

The southern part of the country receives a lot of rain; hence the rainy season is divided into two parts. The first is called *pravṛiśht* and the second, the rainy season. The northern part has a shorter rainy season but a longer winter which is divided into two: *hemaṇt* and *shishir*.

Due to the effects of *visarg* and *āadan* periods, the body loses weight at the end of *āadan* and beginning of *visarg*, during both the periods, physical strength and weight are neither gained nor lost. At the end of *visarg*, the body tends to gain strength. Taking into account all such seasonal variations, *Ayuṛved* recommends different food and living habits for different seasons[385].

Winter (*Hemaṇt* and *Shishir*)

These periods are the best as far as health is considered. The body gains maximum strength at this time[386]. Shorter days and longer nights ensure that the body gets more rest and a longer time for digestion. The body gets increased nourishment and hunger also increases. Due to sharpened digestive power, heavy and excess food is also quickly absorbed.

Staying hungry, or eating dry and inadequate in this season is harmful. In the absence of food, the strengthened digestive power attacks and destroys the essential digestive juices leading to an aggravation of *vāyu dosha*, which is characteristically cold and dry[387].

---

383. *Tatra raviṛbhāabhirāadadāanō jagataḥ ṣnēhaṃ vāayanaṣṭēeyra*
Rōokṣāaṣçhōpaśōṣayaṇtaḥ śiśiravasaṇtgrēemēṣu
yathāakamaṃ rāukṣyamutpāadyaṇtē rōokṣāana rasāaritakta kaṣāaya
Kaṭukāanṣçhāabhivaṛdhayaṇtō ṇriṇāaṃ dāuṛbalyamāavahaṇti *(Ch. Su. 6/6)*
Śēetāanśuḥ kḷēdayatyuṛvēe vivaṣwāanṣōoṣaya ṭyāapi
Tāavubhāavapi sanṣritya vāayuḥ pāalayati prajāaḥ *(Su. Sū 6/8)*

384. *Visaṛgaṣtu sāumyaḥ Taṣmiṇnapi kāalamāaṛgamēghavāataṿaṛṣāabihata*
Ṗrabhāavē dakṣiṇaayanagē5ṛkē Śaśiniḥ çhāavyāahatablē śiśirāabhiṛbhāabhiḥ
Śaśvadāapyāayamāanē māahēṇdra salila praśāanṭasanṭāapē jagtyarōokṣāa
rasāaḥ pravaṛdhaṇtē aṃla lavaṇa madhiraḥ yathāakramaṃ balaṃ
çhopaçhēeyēeyētē ṇriṇāamiti *(A.S. Sū. 4/7)*

385. *Āadāavaṇtē ça dāuṛbalyaṃ visaṛgāadāanaynriṇriṇāam*
Maḍhyē maḍhya balaṃ, ṭwaṇtē śṛēṣṭhamagrē çha niṛdiśēṭ *(Ch. Sū 6/8)*
Hēmaṇṭā śiśirē çhāagrayaṃ visaṛgāadāanayōṛbalaṃ
Śaraḍvaṣaṇtayōṛmaḍhyaṃ hēenaṃ ṿaṛṣāa nidāaghayōḥ *(A.Su. 4/8)*

386. *Dēhō ṣmāaṇō viśaṇtō5ṇtaḥ śēetē śēetāanitāahatāaḥ*
Jatharē pinḍitōṣmāaṇaṃ prabalaṃ kuṛvatē5nalaṃ *(A.S. Su. 4/12)*

♦ Wholesome Diet

A diet that is greasy, sweet, salty, sour and nutritious is best during winter. The following food items must be a part of the winter diet: *Ghēe*, butter, oil, milk, rice-milk pudding, pulse (*Black gram*)-milk pudding, *miśhri*,thickened sweetened milk *(rabri)*, cream, honey with cold milk, sugarcane juice, gruel, sweet made of flour/rice *(halwa)*, sweetened and preserved apple , gooseberry, *amla,* sweets made with *piṭthi* and dry fruits, sprouted pulses, bread of wheat or gram flour , cornflakes, new rice, apple, gooseberry, oranges, *parwal* (tricisanthes diocia), brinjal, cauliflower, cabbage, *jimicand (Anorphophallus Campanulatus)*, ripe red tomatoes, carrot, beans, peas, spinach, fenugreek leaves, *bathua (chenopodium album)*, all other green leafy vegetables, dry ginger, warm water and hot foods are good for health[388].

♦ Wholesome Living

One should stay happy and tension-free. One must wake-up before sunrise; complete all morning activities like cleaning of bowels, bathing etc., and then go for a brisk walk in the fresh air. On returning and resting for a while, one must exercise and do *Yog*. Exercising tones the body, keeps it strong and helps to digest food. Body massage with oil and medicated paste (turmeric *ubtan*) and oiling hair should be a part of one's routine. Massaging with mustard oil keeps the skin beautiful and disease-free, and cures boils and pimples. Oil medicated with camphor cures arthritis and joint pain[389]. Oil massages should be followed by *ubtan*. Exercising can precede or follow body massages.

During winters the skin becomes dry. Exposure to cold can cause cold, fever and pneumonia. Cold winds must be avoided as they can cause cough, asthma, arthritis, itching, etc. One must try and stay in warm places. Heavy, warm woolen clothes and quilts should be used. Sitting in the sun and near a fire helps to keep the body warm. Heat from the sun should be taken on the back,

---

387. Visaṛgē balināaṃ prāayaḥ ṣwāabhāavāadiguru ķśamaṃ
Ḅrihaṇāaṇyaṇnapāanāani yōjayēṭ taṣya yuķtayē
Anindhanō5nyathāa sēedēdatyudēerṇatayāa5thavāa
Dhāatōonapi pachēdaṣya tataṣṭēṣāam ķśayāanmaruṭ
Tējaḥ sahaçharaḥ kupyēçhheetaḥ śeetēviśēṣataḥ *(A.S. Sū 4/13-14)*

388. Atō himē bhajēṭ ṣnigdhāaṇ ṣwāaḍbalaṃ lavaṇāaṇ rasāaṇ *(A.S. Sū 4/15)*
Māaṣēķṣuķśeera viķriti vaśāa taila navāudanāaṇ *(AS. Su. 4/17)*

389. Vyāayāamōḍvaṛtanāaḅhyaṇga ṣwēdadhōomāaṇjanāatapāaṇ *(A.S.Sū. 4/17)*
Sukhōdakaṃ śāuchavidhāu bhōomigaṛbhagrihāaṇicha
Sāaṇrgāarayāanāaṃ śayyāaṃ çha kuthakaṃbalasaṇṣkritāaṃ *(AS. Su 4/18)*
Kuṃkuṃēnāanuliṗtāaṇgō5guruṇāa guruṇāa5pi vāa
Laghuśṇāiḥ ṗravṛitaḥ ṣwaṗyāaṭ kāalē dhōopāadhi vāasitaḥ *(A.S. Su 4/19)*
Pēenāaṇganāaṇgasaṇsaṛganivāaritahimāanilah *(A.S.Su. 4/20)*
Śaradāani çha māalyāani vāasāasi vimalāani çha
Śaraṭkāalē ṗraśaṣyaṇtē ṗradōṣē çheṇdurśmayaḥ *(Ch. Su. 6/48)*

while that from fire should be received from the front. Room heaters can be used to warm the rooms. Sexual activity can be prolific in this season. Milk and *vrishay* substances should be taken at night.

♦ *Unwholesome Food and Habits*

Light, dry, *vāyu*-dominant, bitter, pungent and astringent foods, and stale and cold drinks must be avoided. Sour items like tamarind, dried mango powder (*amchōor*), sour curd, mango pickle should also be, as far as possible, avoided[390].

One must refrain from staying up late at night, getting up late, laziness, escaping work and exercise, staying hungry, bathing too much, trying to bear too much cold, eating late at night and sleeping immediately after eating are unwholesome habits. Those who use myrobalan *harad* as elixir/for rejuvenation should take half a teaspoon of myrobalan *harad* with ginger powder during winter and, half a of myrobalan *harad* teaspoon powder with lukewarm water during severe winter[391].

♦ Difference between *Hemaṇt* and *Shishir*

The weather during both is similar[392]. During mild winter the movement of the sun is in the southern direction, making food and medicinal preparations smooth, sweet and nourishing. There is no *dosha* aggravation during this period. During extreme winter, the sun moves towards the north causing the temperature to fall further and increasing dryness. The coldness, heaviness and sweetness of food acquired during this period, aggravates the *kapha dosha*. Therefore, one must eat only appropriate food, protect oneself from cold and stay in a warm place during extreme winter. Cold and light foods and fasting must be avoided.

If appropriate diet and living habits are adopted during winters, the body can acquire so much strength as to keep fit and healthy throughout the year .

♦ Spring

Spring is the most pleasant of all seasons. A profusion of flowers and natural fragrances all around characterizes this season, which sees winter transforming into summer. During spring the weather is mild and pleasant, the days are warm and nights are cool[393].

♦ Effects on the Body

The intensity of the sunrays increases gradually but steadily during this season. The warmth

---

390. *Vaṛjayēdatṛapāanani vāatalāani laghōoni ćha*
Ṛravāataṃ ṛramitāa55hāaramuḍmaṇthaṃ himāagamē (Ch. Sū 6/18)

391. *Harēetakēe manuśyāaṇāaṃ māatēva hitakāariṇēe*
Kadāachiṭ kuṛyatē māatāa nōdaraṣthāa harēetakēe (Bha. Pra.)
Ģrēe ṣmē tulyagudāamaṃ suśāiḍhvaynvāyuvāaṃ medhāavanaḍwāaṃbarē
Sāaṛdha śaṛkarayāa śāraḍhamalayāa śuṣṭhayāa tuṣāarāagamē
Piṛpaṭyāa śiśirē vasaṇtasamayē kṣāuḍrēṇa sanyōjitāaṃ
Rāajaṇ ṛrāaṛya harēetakēemipa rujō naṣyaṇtu tē śaṭravaḥ (Bh. Vi. Ni.)

392. *Śiśirē śēetamadhikaṃ mēdhamāarutavaṛṣajaṃ*
Rāukṣyaṃ ćhāadāanajaṃ taṣmāaṭ kāaryaḥ pōoṛvōśdhikaṃ vidhiḥ (A.S.Su 4/20)

from the sun melts the *kapha* accumulated in the body during winters. This aggravates it causing cough, cold, sinus, asthma, tonsils, irritation in the throat, decreased digestive power and a nauseous feeling. Moisture and unctuousness decline due to increased warmth of the sun and decrease cool of the moon. This makes body lose weight. Hence one must be particular about diet. Eating sour, sweet and salty foods only aggravates *kapha* further[394].

♦ Wholesome Diet

Diet should be fresh, light and easily digestible. A bitter, juicy, pungent and astringent diet is recommended. The following food items are beneficial during spring:

Rotis (bread) made of green gram, chick pea and barley flour, old wheat and rice, barley, chick pea, mustard seed, sprouted chick peas buttered *roti* and bread, green vegetables and their soup, mustard oil, bitter gourd, garlic, spinach, banana flowers, *Amorphophallus Campanulatus (jimicand)*, radish, new leaves of neem, dried ginger, Indian fig, black pepper, myrobalan *(harad)*, beleric myrobalan *(bahedā)*, gooseberry, roasted and parched rice, Khus-Khus *(khus)* water, lemon, seasonal fruits and honey. Plenty of water should be consumed during spring[395]. Water with ginger juice or honey is nourishing. *Vaman* (induced vomiting) and *harad* powder mixed with honey, reduces *kapha*.

Light exercises should be done regularly. Morning walk, massage with oil and medicated pastes followed by warm water

---

393. Vasaṇtē dakṣ̣inō vāayurāatāamṛakiraṇō raviḥ *(A.S. Sū 4/21)*
Nava pṛavāalaṭwakḥ patrāaḥ pāadapāaḥ kakubhō5malāaḥ
Kinśukāaśōkaçhōotāadivanarāajivirāajitāaḥ *(A.S. Su. 4/22)*
Kōkilāalikulāalāapakōlāahalāakulāaḥ *(A.S.Sū 4/23)*

394. Śiśirē saṇchitaḥ ślēṣmāa dinakṛiḍbhāabhirēeritaḥ *(A.S.Sū 4/23)*
Tadāa pṛabāadhāmāanō5gnim̩ rōgāaṇ prakurutē bahōoṇ *(A.S.Sū 4/24)*

395. Atā5ṣminṣtēekṣ̣na vamana dhōoma gaṇḍōoṣanāavanam̩ *(A.S.Sū 4/24)*
Ṿyayāamōḍnaṛtana kṣ̣āuḍrayavagōdhōomajāaṇgagalāaṇ
Sēvētā suḥriduḍyāanayuvatēeṣ̣ẹha manōramāaḥ *(A.S.Sū 4/25)*
Ṣnāataḥ ṣwalaṇkṛitaḥ ṣragvēe chaṇḍanāagururuṣitaḥ
Vichiṭrāamaṭra viṇyaṣṭāaṇ sahakāarōṭpatāaṇkitāaṇ *(26)*
Nirjadāaṇṣ̣çhāasavāariṣ̣ta sēedhu māaṛḍvēe kamāadhavāaṇ
ḳwathim̩ muṣtaśuthayam̩bu sāarāam̩bhaḥ kṣ̣āuḍḍravāari vāa *(Guruśēetadivāaṣwapṇa)*
Ṣnigdhāam̩lamadhurāaṇṣṭyajēṭ *(A. S. Su 4)*
Atā5ṣminṣtēekṣ̣na vamana dhōoma gaṇḍōoṣanāavanam̩ *(A.S.Sū 4/24)*
Ṿyayāamōḍnaṛtana kṣ̣āuḍrayavagōdhōomajāaṇgagalāaṇ
Sēvētā suḥriduḍyāanayuvatēeṣ̣ẹha manōramāaḥ *(A.S.Sū 4/25)*
Ṣnāataḥ ṣwalaṇkṛitaḥ ṣragvēe chaṇḍanāagururuṣitaḥ
Vichiṭrāamaṭra viṇyaṣṭāaṇ sahakāarōṭpatāaṇkitāaṇ *(26)*
Nirjadāaṇśchāasavāariṣ̣ta sēedhu māaṛḍvēe kamāadhavāaṇ
ḳwathim̩ muṣtaśuthayam̩bu sāarāam̩bhaḥ kṣ̣āuḍḍravāari vāa *(Guruśēetadivāaṣwapṇa)*
Ṣnigdhāam̩lamadhurāaṇṣṭyajēṭ *(A. S. Su 4)*

bath, medicated smoking and putting *kohl* in the eyes are beneficial. Excretory organs should be properly cleaned while bathing. Using fragrances like camphor, sandalwood, *kumkum* after bathing keeps one fresh. Caps and umbrellas must be used to shield against the sunrays whose intensity increases gradually during this season[396]. Spending time in open areas, gardens and parks enjoying the natural beauty calms the mind and evokes a sense of well-being[397]. One can also bath again in the evening during spring.

♦ Unwholesome Diet and Habits

Avoid heavy, oily, sour, sweet and cold foods. Heavy items like grains, *uḍad* pulse, thickened sweetened milk *(rabadi)*, cream and dates etc. are also best avoided. Sleeping under open sky, and exposure to cold and sun is harmful[398].

♦ Summer

Intense heat during this season absorbs all moisture and oil. Temperature shoots up increasing dryness and dullness. This is the peak of the *āadan* period. Everything, from humans, animals, vegetation, to water bodies is affected[399].

♦ Effects on Body

Moisture, oil and coolness are required in great quantities to keep oneself healthy and strong. Because there is a decrease in the quantities of these things in summer, the body, like vegetation, begins to dry. There is a corresponding weakening of all seven *dhātus* in the body, leading to weight loss. Sweating increases. So does thirst. Excessive water intake dilutes the acid in the intestines, increasing chances of loose motions and nausea. Aggravated *piṭta* increases susceptibility to excessive thirst, fever, burning sensations, bleeding (from nose etc.), dizziness, headache, etc. To avoid falling prey to these ailments, and to maintain body weight and strength during summer, *Ayurved* recommends the following diet and life-style habits.

---

396. *Eētēḥ praśamaṇam balayaṃ gupṭyāavaranāśankaram*
Dharmāanilarajō5ṃbuḍhnaṃ çhhaṭradhāarnamuçhyatē *(Ch. Sū 5/101)*

397. *Kakumēnāanuliptāangō5guruṇāa, guruṇāa5pi vāa* *(A.S. Sū 4/19)*

398. *Guru śēeta divāa ṣwapna ṣnighāamla madhurāanṣtyajeṭ* *(A.S.Su. 4/28)*

399. *Taṭra raviṛbhāabhirāadadāanō jagataḥ ṣnēhaṃ vāayavaṣṭēevra*
-rōokśāaṣçhōpaśōṣayanṭaḥ śiśiravasanṭagrēe ṣmēṣu yathāakramam
rāukṣyaṃ uṭpāadayanṭō rōokśāanraśāanṣṭikṭakaṣāayakaṭukāan
-ṣçhāabhivardhayanṭō ṇriṇāaṃ dāurbalyamāavahanṭi *(Ch. Su. 6/6)*
Tāa aivāuṣadhayō nidāahē niṣsāarāa rōokśa atimāatram laghvyō
bhavanṭyāapa ṣçha tāa upyujyamāanāaḥ sōoryapratāapōpaśōṣitadēhāahāam
dēhināaṃ rāukṣyāallaghuṭwāadwāiśadāaçhçha vāayōḥ sanchayamāapāadyanti
Gṛēeṣmē tēekśṇāanṣurāadiṭyo māarutōṇāuritō5sukhaḥ *(Su. Su. 6/13)*
bhōoṣtapṭāa saritaṣṭanvyō diśaḥ prajwalitāa iva *(Su. Sū 6/31)*
Diśō jwalanṭi bhōomiṣçha māarutō nāiṛirtaḥ sukhaḥ
Pavanāatapasanṣwēdāirjanṭavō jwaritāa iva *(A.S.Su. 4/29)*

♦ Wholesome Diet And Living[400]

Light, oily, sweet, easily digestible, cold and liquid foods must form a major part of diet in summers. Boiled water, cooled in fridge or earthen pots must be used.

The following food items are recommended: Sugar, *ghēe* (clarified butter), milk, butter milk with sugar, salt and roasted cumin in the mornings and afternoons (avoid at night), old and fermented barley, *arhar* pulse, *chāulāi (amaranthus)*, bitter gourd, *bathua (chenopodium album)*, *parwal (tricisanthes diocia)*, ripe tomatoes, unpeeled potatoes, unripe banana fruit curry, drum-stick, horse-radish, onion, white pumpkin, mint, lemon, polished green gram, *arhar* and *masoor* pulses, watermelon, muskmelon, sweet mango, oranges, grapes, *kakdi (cucumis utilissimus)*, mulberry, *faalsa* (berry of *grewia asiatica)*, pomegranate, preserved and sweetened gooseberry, raisins, dates in liquids, sweetened fresh lime juice, juice of green unripe mango, sherbets, sweetened buttermilk, wood-apple sherbet, sweet diluted coarse grain flour (barley, gram etc.), *thandai* (cooling drink containing ground spices, seeds etc.), sandalwood, *khaskhas* (a kind of poppy seed) and rose sherbets, sugarcane, apple and sweet orange juices, water cooled with camphor and trumpet flowers *(bignonia sauvolens)*, coconut water, milk with *ghēe* and sugar, buffalo milk, water cooled in moonlight, ice-cream etc. *Arhar* pulse is dry. A little *ghēe* and cumin seeds should be added to it. Myrobalan should be taken only with jaggery.

During summer, the quantity of diet should be reduced and food must be properly chewed. Only freshly cooked and warm food should be eaten. Prolonged refrigeration and reheating should be avoided. Eating foods refrigerated for a very long time is harmful. Water cooled in earthen pots is better than refrigerated water.

Walking must be done under the cover to avoid exposure to sun. Rooms should be adequately cooled. The sleeping room should have access to moonlight and fresh air. Applying sandalwood paste on the body and wearing pearl jewellery is good. Bed should be covered with banana, *kalhāar*, lotus stalk, and lotus leaves[401]. Light coloured cotton clothes must be worn. To prevent heatstroke, exposure to sun and hot dry winds, good

---

400. *Mayukhāiṛjagataḥ ṣnēhaṃ grēeṣmē pēpēeyate raviḥ*
Swāaduśēetaṃ ḍravaṃ ṣnigdhaṃ aṇapāanaṃ tadāa hitaṃ
Śēetaṃ saśaṛkaraṃ maṇthaṃ jāaṇgalāaṇṃrigapakṣ́iṇaḥ
gritaṃ payaḥ saśāalyaṇnaṃ bhajaṇ grēeṣmē na sēedati **(Ch. Sū 27-28)**
Āadaṭṭē jagataḥ ṣnēhāaṇṣtadāadiṭyō ḅhṛiśaṃ yataḥ
Ṿyāayāamāatapa kaṭwaṃlalavaṇōṣ̄ṇaṃ tyajēdataḥ **(A.Su Sū 4/32)**
Maḍyaṃ na sēṿyaṃ ṣwalpaṃ vāa sēṿyaṃ subahu vāari vāa
Aṇyathāa śōṣaśāithilyāahamōhāaṇ karōti taṭ **(A. S. Sū 4/33)**
Nava ṃṛiḍbhāajanaṣthāani ḥvaghāani surabhēeṇi ċha
Pāanakāani samaṇthāani sitāaḍyāani himāani ċha **(A.S. Sū 4/34)**
Ṣwāaduśēetaṃ ḍravaṃ ċhāaṇṇaṃ jāaṇgalāaṇṃrigapakṣ́iṇaḥ
Śāalikṣ́ēera grita ḍrāakṣ́āa nāarikērāaṃbu śaṛkarāah **(A.S. Sū 4/35)**

shoes, protective headgear and umbrellas must be used. A cool glass of water before venturing out in the sun is helpful. Carrying an onion in the pocket also helps. If one requires staying awake after 10 pm, a glass of cool water every now and then should be taken. It keeps the *vāyu* and *kapha doshas* in control, and prevents constipation[402].

Dinner should be early, light and easily digestible. If possible, a couple of times a week, it should be restricted to only gruel. Afternoon siesta in this season is not harmful.

♦ Unwholesome Diet and Living

The quantity of foods that are hot, sour, bitter, salty, dry and astringent should be kept to the minimum. Heavy, fried, hot, spicy and stale foods, *uṛad* pulse, garlic, mustard, stale and sour curd, honey, brinjal, ice etc. should be completely avoided. (Honey can be used as medicine). Fast foods like *chāat*, sweets made of condensed milk, and *uṛad* pulse preparations are damaging. Drinking too much water at one go weakens the digestive system. A glass of water at regular intervals is advised. Sudden exposure to contrasting temperatures is dangerous. For example, walking out into blazing sun from a cold room, or drinking chilled water immediately after being in the sun. Water should be taken after the sweat has dried and the body temperature has cooled off a bit. It is a good idea to mix refrigerated water with normal water kept at room temperature. Alcoholic drinks must be completely avoided. Those who are addicted to them, must dilute the drinks as much as possible.

The following food and living habits must also be avoided during summers :-

Staying awake too long in the night, (as the nights are short in summers) prolonged exposure to sun, going out without covering head, remaining hungry and thirsty for long, over exercising, avoiding elimination of urine and stool, and sexual activity (it should be reduced to once a fortnight)[403].

---

401. *Divāa śēetagihē niḍrāaṃ niśi çhanḍrāaṇśuśēetalē*
Bhajēchçhaṇḍanadigdhāaṇgaḥ pravāatē harṃyamaṣtakē
Ṿyajanāiḥ pāaṇisaṇsparāiśçhiṇdanōdakaśēetalāih
Sēvyamāanō bhajēdāaṣyaṃ mukṭāamaṇivibhuṣitaḥ
Ḳāanāani çha śēetāaṇi jalāani kusumāani cha (Ch. Su. 6/30-32)
Tāalavṛinṭāanilāaṇ hāarāaṇ ṣrijaḥ sakamaloṭ palāah
Taṇvēemriṇāala valayāaḥ kāaṇṭāaśchaṇdaruṣitāaḥ
Sarāaṇsi vāapēeḥ saritah kāananāani himaani cha
Surabhēeṇi niṣēvēta vāasāaṇsi Sulaghōoni cha (A.S. Su. 4/36-37)
Niṣpatadyaṇtrasalilē ṣwapyāadadhāarāagrihē divāa
Rāatrāu çhāakāaśatalakē sugaṇdhikhsumāaṣṭritē (A.S. Su 4/38)

402. *Maḍyamalpaṃ na vāa pēyamathavāa subahōodakaṃ*
Lavaṇāaṃlḳakaṭṣ̄ṇāani ṿyāayāanmaṃ chāaṭra varjayāt (Ch. Su. 6/20)
Kaṛpōoraçhaṇḍavāaṛdrāaṇgō viralāanaṇgasaṇgamaḥ (A.S.Sū. 4/39)

403. *Grēeṣmakāalē niṣēvēt māithunāad viratōnaraḥ* (Ch.su. 6/32)
Karpōoraçhaṇḍanāaṛdrauṇgō viralāanangasaṇgamaḥ (A.S. Su. 4/39)

♦ Rainy Season

Rainy season happens at the commencement of *visarg* period. It is characterized by greenery all around, cloud cover, humidity and an increase in the numbers of mosquitoes and flies.

♦ Effect on the Body

The increased humidity has its effect on the body. It aggravates the *vāta dosha* and weakens the already affected digestive powers. Due to moisture caused by rain, *vata dosh*a increases and digestive power decreases. Digestive power is also affected by the dust and smoke, increased sourness in *jalan* (water and foods stuffs) and gases released from the earth due to rains[404]. On days that it doesn't rain, the heat increases causing an accumulation of the *piṭta dosha* in the body. Nutritive value of wheat, rice and other food items is reduced. Due to these reasons and increased chances of infection, diseases like malaria, cold, diarrhoea, dysentry, cholera, colitis, *alsak*, arthṛitis, swelling in joints, high blood pressure, pimples, ringworms, itching etc. can be easily contracted[405].

♦ Wholesome Food and Living

Diet during rains must be light, fresh, hot, easily absorbed and one that strengthens digestion. It should be capable of calming *vāyu dosha*. Hence the diet should include, old grains like wheat, barley, *shāali* rice, corn, rice, mustard, linseed, cucumber, gruel, curd, buttermilk, green gram, *arhar* pulse. In vegetables, green gourd, okra (ladies finger), turai (luffa acutangula), tomatoes, mint chutney,[406] vegetable soups, and in fruits apple, banana, pomegranate, pear, blackberry, ripe mangoes, salty dishes made in *ghēe* and oil. Mangoes and milk are particularly beneficial[407]. The mango must be ripe, sweet and fresh. It can cause harm if it is unripe and sour. Drinking milk after eating a mango is nourishing. If this combination can replace a

---

404. *Āadāanaduṛbatē dēhē paḳtāa bhavati duṛbalaḥ*
Sa ṿaṛṣāaṣwanilāadēenāaṃ dōoṣnaibāadhayatē punaḥ *(Ch. Su. 6/33)*
Tadāa55dāanāabatē dēhē meṇdē5gnāu bāadhitē punaḥ *(A.A.AU. 4/42)*

405. *Nabhasi meghāavatate jalapraḳliṇṇāaṃ bhōomāu milaṇnadehāanāaṃ*
Ṗrāaṇināaṃ śēetavāataviṣṭaṃbhitāagnēenāam vidaḥyaṇte
Vidāahāaṭ piṭtasaṇçhayamāapāadayaṇti
Ṿriṣṭibhōovāaṣpatōyāaṃlapāaka duṣṭāīṣçhalāadibhiḥ *(A.S.Su. 4/43)*

406. *Pāanabhōjansaṇskāarāaṇ pṛāayaḥ ḳṣāuḍrāaṇvitāaṇ bhajeṭ*
Ṿyaḳtaṃlalavaṇaṣnēhaṃ vāatavṛṣāakulē5hani
Viśeśēetē bhōḳtaṿuyaṃ varṣāaṣwanilaśāaṇtayē
Agnisaṇraḳśaṇavatāaṃ yavagōdhōonaśāalayaḥ
Purāaṇāa jāaṇgalāiṛmāasāiṛbhojyāa yoṣāiṣçha saṇḳritālḥ *(Ch.Su. 6/31-38*

407. *Piṭāanilakaraṃ bāalaṃ piṭtalaṃ baḍdhakēsaraṃ*
Ḥridyaṃ vaṛṇakaraṃ ruçhyaṃ reḳtamāaṃsabalapradaṃ
Kaṣāayānurasaṃ ṣwāadu vāatahunaṃ ḅraṇhaṇaṃ guru
Piṭtavirōdhi sopaṇḳwāaṃraṃ śuḳravivaṛdhanaṃ *(Su.Su. 46/152-153)*
Āaṃraṣya pallauōruçhyaḥ kapharpiṭtavinaśanaṃ *(Bha. pea 18)*

meal, the body gains strength and stability. Similarly regular use of ripe blackberry heals boils and pimples, burning, and skin and urinary diseases[408]. Roasted corn is easily digested if followed by buttermilk. Diluted curd with clove, *trikatu* (dry ginger, black pepper and long pepper), rock salt, thymol, and black salt keeps digestion strong. Garlic *chuṭney,* and honey in water also prove beneficial. To calm *vāyu* and *kapha doshas* in this season, bitter, sour and alkaline substances should be taken. Sour, salty and oily foods calm *vāyu* especially when the weather cools down due to heavy rains and winds. Myrobalan, in this season, should be taken with rock salt. Cleanliness of water should be ascertained before consumption. It should be boiled and cooled. It can also be treated with *tulsi* leaves and a pinch of alum powder. Filters and other modern techniques are very helpful. Honey can be mixed in this purified and cool water. Massaging with oil and medicated pastes, and fomentation is beneficial[409]. Clothing should be clean and light[410]. Places exposed to humidity and draught must not be used for sleeping. Food must be taken only when hungry. Dinner should be early. Care should be taken to avoid being bitten by mosquitoes. Surrounding areas should be regularly cleaned and stagnant water should be sprayed with insecticides[411].

♦ Unwholesome Diet and Living

Pulse Leafy vegetables, cold and dry foods, gram, kidney bean, *uṛad*, barley, peas, *masoor* pulse (lens esculenta), millet, potato, jack fruit, water cress, bitter gourd and parched grain gruel are harmful in this season. When the rains are light, *piṭta* increases. At such times sour, fried, eatables made from gram flour, hot and spicy, stale and other *piṭta* aggravating foods should be avoided. According to a popular saying, milk in *shrāavan* (july-august), buttermilk in *bhāaḍrpad* (mid-august to mid September), bitter gourd in *ḳwāar* (September-October), and curd in *kāṛtik* (October-November) are to be avoided. Sleeping in the afternoon or in the sun, exposure to sun, excessive sexual activity, walking and exercising too much is dangerous[412]. Heavy diet, eating frequently and without hunger is also detrimental. Curd

---

408. *Ḉrāahēe kaaṣāyaṣtaṇmajjāaa viśeṣāṇmadhumehahāa* ***(mōolaphala vaṛg Nir)***
Jambōo kaṣaayamadhurāa śṛamapiṭtadāahakaṇthāaṛṭi
śōṣaśamanēe ḳrimidōṣahaṇtrēe
Ṣwāasāatisāarakaphakāasavināaśinē ḉhaviṣṭaṃbhinēe bhavati
rōchanaapāachanēe cha ***(Ra Ni)***

409. *Pibēṭ ḳxāuḍrāaṇvita chāalpaṃ māaḍhuēekāariṣṭamaṃbu vāa*
Māahēḍraṃ taptaśēetaṃ vāa kāupaṃ sāarasunmēua vāa ***(Ch.Su. 6/39)***

410. *Ṗragharṣōḍvaṛtana ṣnāanagaṇḍhamāalyaparō bhavēṭ*
Laghuśudhāaṃbarah ṣthāanaṃ bhajēdaḳlēdi vaaṛṣikaṃ ***(Ch.Sū 6/40)***
Ṗragharṣōḍvaṛtana ṣnāanadhọomagaṇḍhāaguruṗriyaḥ
Yāayāaṭkarēṇu muḳhyāa bhiṣḉhitra ṣṭragvaṣṭrabhōoṣitaḥ ***(A.S. Su. 4/48)***

411. *Nadēejalōdamaṇthāaḥaḥ ṣwapṇāatiḍṛavamāithunaṃ*
Ṭuṣāarapāadaḉharaṇa ṿyāayāamāaṛkakarāaṇṣṭyajeṭ ***(A.S. Su 4/49)***

and buttermilk should be completely avoided. Wet and damp clothes or bed should not be used. The body, especially joints and places with tender skin should be kept dry. Vegetables and fruits must be thoroughly washed before use. Medication for loose motions should not be taken if it is cloudy outside. Ice cubes or other effective medicines help relieve prickly heat.

One can enjoy the rainy season to the fullest if the above diet and lifestyle tips are followed.

♦ Autumn

This season is characterized by presence of clear and beautiful clouds, stronger and pleasant moonlight that evokes contentment and lends purity to rivers, lakes and ponds. Sour essence becomes predominant in vegetation and herbs[413].

♦ Effects on Body

During rains the body becomes accustomed to cool weather. In autumn the sun shines with full intensity, aggravating the *piṭta dosha* that accumulates in the body during the rains[414]. This corrupts the blood. As a result, there is an increase in *piṭta* and blood related disorders like fever boils and pimples, rashes, throat infection, itching etc. Being the middle of *visarg* period, physical strength is neither too high nor too low.

♦ Wholesome Food and Living

Ghēe and pungent foods should be used to deal with vitiated *piṭta*. Other food items that help are those that are sweet, light, cool, pungent and digestible *shāali*[415] rice, green gram, wheat, barley, boiled milk, curd, butter, *ghēe*, cream, *shrikhand*. In vegetables *Chenopodium album (chāulāyi bathūa)*, green gourd, *Lufta acutangula (torai)*, cauliflower, raddish, spinach, soya bean, gooseberry, beans *(sem)*, pomegranate, watercress, fig, and lotus seed are good in this season. Gooseberry should be eaten with sugar. Pungent things should be cooked in clarified butter. Water treated with sun-rays and moonlight should be used. Such water is considered as good as nectar due to the effect of the star Canopus. It should also be used for bathing and swimming[416]. *Āchāṛya Çharak* considered this water a "*haṇsodak*". Myrobalan in this season should be taken in the powdered form mixed with honey, sugar candy or jaggery[417].

---

412. Udamaṇthaṃ divāaṣwapṇaṃ avaśyāayaṃ nadēejalaṃ
Vyāayāamamāatapaṃ chāiva vyavāayaṃ çhāaṭra varjayēṭ *(Ch. Su 6/35-36)*

413. Śaradi vyōma śubhrāabhraṃ kiṇchiṭ paṇkaṇkitāa mahēe
Prakāaśakāaśasapṭāaḥrikumudāa śaaliśaalinēe *(A.S. Su 4/50)*
Tapṭāanāaṃ saṇçhçhitaṃ pōoṛva tadāa piṭtaṃ prakupyati *(A. S. Su. 4/53)*

414. Vaṛṣāaśēetōçhitāaṇganāaṃ sahasāivāṛṛkaraṣmibhiḥ
Tapṭāanāaṃāaçhitaṃ piṭtaṃ prāayaḥ śaradi kupyati *(Ch. Su. 6/41)*

415. Taṇṇāaṇnapāanāṃ madhuraṃ laghuśēetaṃ satiḳtakaṃ
Piṭṭapraśamaṇaṃ śevyaṃ māaṭrayāa suprakāaṇkitāiḥ
Śaalēeṇ sayavagōdhōomāaṇ śēvyāanāahuṛghanāaṭyayē *(Ch. Su. 6/42)*
Śēetaṃ laghvaṃnapāanaṃ çha kaṣāayaṣwāadutiḳtaṃ
Śāali ṣaṣṭikgōdhōomayavamuḍgasitāamadhu *(A.S.Su 4/55)*

Enema and blood letting calms the vitiated blood and *piṭṭa*. This protects against corresponding ailments[418]. Seasonal flowers should be used for adornment. Walking, sleeping or resting in the moonlight is beneficial.

♦ **Unwholesome Food And Diet**

Avoiding oily foods, oil (mustard), buttermilk, anise, garlic, brinjal, bitter gourd, asafoetida, black pepper, long pepper, dishes made of *Black gram* pulse, sour foods like *kadhi*, alkaline drinks, strong alcoholic substances, curd and salty food items is beneficial in autumn. Eating when not hungry is harmful. One should protect onself from exposure to sun, dew and west wind. Excessive exercise and sexual activity is also harmful[419].

Suitable Diet in Brief	
Winter and Rains	Sweet, sour, salty, unctuous and hot foods.
Spring	Pungent, bitter, astringent, dry and hot foods.
Autumn	Sweet, pungent, astringent, dry and cool foods.
Summer	Sweet, unctuous, and cool foods.

Though food with all taste essences should be eaten during all seasons, the quantity of foods listed above should be increased according to the seasons mentioned.

It is important to remember that diet should not be changed abruptly with the change in

---

416. *Divāasōoryāaṇśusaṇtaptaṃ niśi chaṇdrāaṇśuśēetalaṃ*
    Kāalēṇa pakvaṃ nirdōśa agaṣṭyēnāaviṣeekṛitaṃ
    Haṅsḍakamiti khyāataṃ śāaradaṃvimalaṃ śuchi
    Ṣṇāanapāanāavagāahēṣu śaṣyatē tadyathāa5ṃritaṃ
    Śāaradāani cha māalyāani vāasāaṇsi vimlāani cha
    Saraṭkāalē praśaṣyaṇtē pradōśē chenduraṣmayaḥ   (Ch. Sū 6/46-48)
417. *Sēvēt chaṇdrakiraṇāaṇ pradōśaṃ sāughamāaśritaḥ*
    Triptidaḍhyāata pakṣāarvasāailapurō5nīlāaṇ   (A.S. Su 4/59)
418. *Tiktaṣya sarpiṣaḥ pāanaṃ virēkō raktamōkṣaṇam*   (Ch. Su. 6/42)
    Śaṣṭaṃ tiktahaviḥ pāanaṃ virēkōṣṣraṣrutih sadāa
    Śēetaṃ laghkaṇṇ apāanaṃ cha kaṣwāayaṣwāadutiktakaṃ   (A.S. Su 4/54)
419. *Āatapaṣya cha varjanaṃ*
    Vasāaṃ tailamava śyāayamāudakāaṇōopamāamiṣam
    Kṣāaraṃ dadhi divāaṣwapnaṃ prāagvāataṃ chāaṭra varjayēṭ   (Ch. Su 6/44-515)

seasons[420]. This will cause imbalance and disharmony in the body leading to ailments. Food and lifestyle habits should be modified gradually. The time between two seasons is *Yamdrashtra* according to *Achāṛya*, especially the last 8 days of *kārtik* and the first 8 days of *aghan*. During this period all rules must be followed strictly.

4. Suppression of Natural Urges[421]

It has been commonly observed that avoiding eating when hungry leads to a sudden drop in energy levels. Similarly not quenching thirst makes one feel lifeless and giddy. Avoiding passing urine or stool on experiencing the urge to do so, leads to pain in the bladder and formation of gas. The most natural conclusion of these observations is that suppression of natural urges is harmful. There are other natural urges in addition to the ones mentioned above. These urges are felt by all conscious beings. Timely satisfaction of these urges is paramount to good health. Postponing or ignoring them can lead to various kinds of ailments[422].

There are13 main urges listed in the *Ayuṛved*

1. Urination
2. Defecation
3. Sexual desire
4. Flatulence
5. Sneezing
6. Vomitting
7. Eructation(belching)
8. Yawning
9. Hunger
10. Thirst
11. Weeping (tears)
12. Breathing and
13. Sleep.

Suppression of **Natural urges** leads to the following :

- **Urination**[423] – pain in bladder and genital organs, dysuria, headache,

---

420. *Ṛitusaṇdhiḥ - Riṭwōraṇṭyāadisapṭāahāadṛitusaṇdhiṇritiṣṃritaḥ*
Taṭra pōoṛvō vidhiṣṭyāajyaḥ sēvanēeyō5paraḥ Ḳramāaṭ
Asāaṭṃjāa hi rōgāaḥ ṣyuḥ sahasāa tyāagaśēelanāaṭ (A. S. Su 4/61)
Kāaṛtikaṣya dināaṇyaśṭ̣āavaśṭ̣āa vāagrayaṇaṣya cha
Yamadaṇṣṭ̣rāa samāaḳhyāatāa ṣvialpabhuḳtō hijēevati (Sha. Prakh 2/30)

421. *Rōgāaḥ saṛvēśpi jāayaṇtē vēgōdēeṛaṇadhāaraṇāiḥ*
Vēgadhāaraṇaśēelaṣya ḉha ṣwāaṣthayāasaṇbhavāḥ
Atōvēgadhāaraṇa ṗratiṣēdhēṇa ḉha rōgāanuṭpaṭtiḥ (Aśṭāang Su. Sūśinduṭēekāṇ)

422. *Na vēgāaṇ dhāarayēḍḍhēemāaṇjāatāaṇ mōoṭrapuṛēeṣayōḥ*
Na rētaśō na vāataṣya na ḉḥchhṛdyāaḥ kṣ̣avathōṛna ḉha
Nōḍgāaraṣya na jṛiṃbhāayāa na vēgāaṇ kṣ̣uṭpipāasayōḥ
Navāaśpaṣya na niḍrāayāayāanihṣ̣wāasaṣya ṣ̣ramēṇa ḉha (Ch. Sū 7/3-4)

423 *Vāaṣṭamēhanayōḥ śōolaṃ mōoṭraḳriḉḥchhaṃ śirōrōojāa*
Vināamo vaṇḳṣṇāanaḥaḥ ṣ̣yāaliṇga mōoṭranigrahē
Aṇgabhaṇgāaṣ̣marēevaṣṭimēḍra vaḳśaṇavēdanāaḥ (Ch. Su 7/6)

distension in the lower abdomen. These can be treated with tub- bath, massage, instilling drops of ghee in the nostrils and three types of enema (*āsthapāan*, uttar basti, *anuvāsan*) [424].

- **Defecation** – Avoiding or postponing defecation can cause colic pain, severe headache, constipation, cramps, distension in lower abdomen. Treatments are fomentation, massage, tub-bath, inserting basti in the anus, enema etc. Papaya, green vegetables, fruit juices and other laxatives are helpful. [425,426]

- **Sexual gratification** – pain in the genital organs and testicles, restlessness, cardiac pain, trouble in urine elimination. Treatments are massage, tub-bath, oil-free enema, eating *shāali* rice and milk and using means of means of sexual gratification *(sambhog saadhan)*[427,428].

- **Flatulence** – suppressing the urge to release gas aggravates *vāyu dosha*. It prevents elimination of urine, stool and gas leading to constipation, distension in the lower abdomen, exhaustion and other stomach disorders[429].
Treatment– intake of and massage with oily substances like *ghēe* and oil, fomentation, suppositories enema is beneficial. Consume easily digestive &

---

424. *Ṣwēdāavagāahanāabḥyangāana sarpiṣachāa vapēedakam*
Mōotrēpratihatēkuryāatrividham vaṣtikarma cha **(Ch. Sū 7/7)**
Mōotrajēṣu cha pāane cha prāagbhakṭāachchhsyatēghritam **(A. San. Su. 579)**
Jēerṇāantikaṃ chōṭtamayāa māatṛayāa yōjanāaḍdhidhāaritē
Avapēedakamētachcha sangitaṃ

425. *Pakvāaśayaśirahṣōolaṃ vāatavarchō5pravaṛavartanaṃ*
Pindikōḍdhēṣṭanāadhmāanaṃ purēeṣē syāaḍdhidhāarite **(Ch. Su 7/8)**
Śakṛitahpindi koḍdhēṣṭa pratiśyāaya śirōrōjāah
Ūṛvavāayuh parēekartohridayaṣyōparōdhanaṃ
mukhēna vitpravṛitiśçha **(A. Saṇ Sū 5/6-7)**

426. *Ṣwēdabhyaṇgāavagāahaṣcha vaṛtayōḥ vaṣtikarm cha*
Hitaṃ pratihatē varchasyannapāanaṃ pramāathicha **(Ch. Saṇ Sū 7/9)**

427. *Mēdrē vṛisaṇyōḥ śōolamangamardōhridi vyathāa bhavēṭ*
pratihatē śukre vibadhaṃ mōotramēva cha **(Ch. San Sū 7/10)**
Śukṛāaṭ taṭsravaṇaṃ guhyavēdanāa śvyathajwarāah
hṛiḍvyathāa mōotra saṇgāaṇgabhangavaḍdhyaśmaṣanḍdṭāah **(A. San. Sū 5/23)**

428. *Tatrāabhgaṇgōśkāahṣcha madirāa charaṇāayadhāaḥ*
Śāaliḥ payō nirōḍhṣcha śaṣtaṃ māithunamēva cha **(Ch. Sū 7/11)**

429. *Saṇgōvinmōotra vāatāanāamāadhmāanaṃ vēdanāa klamah*
Jatharē vāatāa jāaṣchāanyē rōgāah syurvāatanigrahāaṭ **(Ch. Su 7/12)**
Adhōvāataṣya rōdhēna gulmōdāavartarōokaklamāldh
Vāatamōotṛakritsaṇgadṛaśyagni vadhahṛidgadāah **(A. San. Su. 5/4)**

430. *Ṣnēhaṣwēdavidhiṣtatra vartayō bhōjanāani cha*
Pāanāani baṣtaya ṣchāiva śaṣtaṃ vāatāanulōmanaṃ **(Ch. Su. 7/13)**

calming drinks[430].

♦ **Vomiting** – Stopping of vomiting causes itching, urticaria, anorexia, oedema, erysipelas (black spots on skin), fever, anaemia, nausea, (*visarp*) and other skin diseases. Treatment – using purgatives and laxatives, medicated smoking, blood-letting, exercising, eating dry foods and drinks.[431,432]

♦ **Sneezing** – Its prevention can cause-headache, paralysis, hemicrania, weakness of sense organs, cervical spondylitis [433].

Treatment- massaging area between head and neck, fomentation, medicated smoking, nasal drops. *Ghee* should be taken after using *vāyu* calming medication and food[434].

♦ **Eructation** – Its obstruction can cause-hiccups, breathlessness, tremors, anorexia, malfunctioning of heart and lungs[435]. Treatment- carminatives, purgation and other remedies to control hiccups[436].

♦ **Yawning**[437] – Its stoppage can cause-convulsions, numbness and tremors in the organs. Treatment – drugs for alleviation of *vāyu* are helpful.

---

431. *Kandōokōthāaruchivyaṇgaśōthapāaṇḍvāamayajwarāaḥ*
     ku ṣṭhaḥrillāasavēesapariçhhiṛdinigrahajāagadāaḥ   (Ch. Su 7/14)
     Visarpakothakuśṭhāakṣikaṇḍōopāaṇḍavāamayāajwarāaḥ
     Sakāasaṣwāashṛrillāasavyamaṇga ṣvayathavō vamēḥ   (A. San. Sū 5/20)

432. *Bhukṭwāa praçhçhhiṛdanaṃ dhamōlaṇghanaṃ raktamōkṣaṇaṃ*
     Rōokṣāannapāanaṃ vyāayāamō virēka ṣçhāatra ṣaṣyatē   (Ch. Su 7/15)
     Gaṇḍōoṣadhōomāahāaharaṃ rōok ṣaṃ bhukṭwāa taduḍwamaḥ
     Vyāayāamaḥ ṣrutirasaṛaṣya śaṣtaṇçhāatra virēçhanaṃ
     Sakṣāaralavaṇaṃ tailamabhyaṇgāartha çha ṣaṣyatē   (A.San. Su. 5/22)

433. *Maṇyāaṣṭaṃbhaḥ śiraḥśōolamaṛditāarlaḍhāavabhēdakāu*
     Iṇḍriyāanāañcha dāuṛbalyaṃ ḳ ṣavathōḥ ṣyāaḍḍhiḍhaaraṇāaṭ   (Ch. Su. 7/16)
     Śirōṛtēeṇḍriyadāuṛbalyamaṇyāaṣṭaṃbhāaṛditaṃ kṣuteḥ   (A.S.Su. 5/12)

434. *Taṭrōṛdhvajaṭrukē5bhyaṇgaḥ śwēdō dhōomaḥ sanāavanaḥ*
     Hitaṃ vāataḍyamāadyaṃ çha gritaṃ çhāutarabhaktikaṃ   (Ch. Su 7/17)
     Tēekṣṇadhōomāanjamāaghrāaṇanāavanāaṛkavilōkanīḥ
     Pravaṛtayēṭ kṣtitiṃ saktāam swēdāavabhyaṇgāu çha śēelayēta
     Yogyaṃ vāataghnamannaṃ cha ghritaṃ çhāuttarabhaktakaṃ   (A. Sam. Su. 5/13)

435. *Hikkāa śwāa5ośruchiḥ kampāavibandhō ṛidayōrasōḥ*   (Ch. Sū 7/18)

436. *Uḍgāaranigrahāaṭtatra hikkāayāaṣtulyāuṣṣadhaṃ*   (Ch.Su 7/18)

437. *Vināamāakṣēpasaṇkōçhāaḥ suptih kampaḥ pravēpaṇaṃ*
     Jrimbhayāa nigrahāaṭtatra sarvaṃ vāataghnamāuṣanaṃ   (Ch. Sū 7/19)
     Jrimbhāayāaḥ kṣavavaḍrōgāaḥ sarvāaṣçhāanilagiḍvidhaḥ   (A. San Sū 5/19)

438. *Kāaṛśyadāuṛbalyavāaivarṇyaṇgamaṛdō5ruçhiṛbhramaḥ*
     Kṣuḍḍhēganigrahāaṭtatra ṣnigadhōṣṇaṃ laghubhōjanaṃ   (Ch. Su. 5/20)

- **Hunger**[438] - Avoiding food when feeling hunging can create problems of-emaciation, weakness, anorexia, giddiness, change in complexion. Treatment – light, hot and unctuous food.
- **Thirst**[439] – Ignoring it can cause-dryness of throat and mouth, deafness, exhaustion, cardiac pain, dizziness etc. Treatment – cold and refreshing drinks.
- **Weeping (tears)**[440] – Avoiding it can cause-rhinitis, eye diseases, heart diseases, anorexia, giddiness. Treatment – sleeping, using alcoholic substances, staying happy.
- **Sleep**[441] – yawning, exhaustion, fatigue, headache, heaviness and giddiness. Treatment – sleeping and resting for the required number of hours. One must consume *vāyu* calming diet and drugs.

Tendencies to Be Kept In Check[442]

Each one of us develops tendencies that are harmful to our self and people around us. These tendencies spring from feelings of greed, fear, anger, sorrow, envy, pride, shamelessness and attachment. To lead a happy and peaceful life, keeping these feelings under check and avoiding acting under their influence is very important. One must also guard against using harsh, abusive and inappropriate language. Acting in a way that disturbs others mentally should be avoided. One must keep away from indulging in activities like stealing or cheating on one's partner. Avoiding these things in thought, word and action leads to a happy and content life. Living a disciplined life where actions are guided by good ideals, leads to enjoyment of the benefits of righteous living, material wealth and sensual gratification[443].

---

439. *Kaṇthāasyaśō ṣobāadḥirya śṛamaḥ sāadō ḥridi vyathāa*
Pipāasāanigṛahāatatra śēetaṃ tarpaṇaṃiśyatē (Ch. Sū 7/21)
Śoṣāaṇgasāadabāadḥiṛagsaṃ mōhabḥramahridagadāah
Ṭri ṣṇāayāa nigrahāaṭtatra śēetaḥsarvōvidhiṛhitaḥ

440. *Pratiśyāayō5kṣirōgaśçhāaruçhiṛbhramaḥ*
Vāaśpanigrahāaṇaṭṭatra ṣwapanō mạdyaṃ priyāaḥ kathāaḥ (Ch.Su 7/22)
Pēenaśāakṣiṛśirōḥridṛuṇgamaṇyāaṣtaṃbhāaruchibḥramāaḥ
Sagulṃāavāśpaṣtatra ṣwapnōmadyaṃ priyāaḥ kathāaḥ (A. Sam. Su. 5/19)

441. *Jriṃbhāa5ṇgamardaṣṭtaṇdrāa ça śirōrōgo5kṣigāuravaṃ*
Nidrāavidhāaraṇāaṭtatra ṣwapnaḥ saṃvāahanāani ça (Ch.Su. 7/23)
Nidrāayāa mohamōorḍhāakṣigāuravāalaṣyajriṃbhikāaḥ
Aṇgamardaśdanṣeha tatrēṣṭaḥ ṣwapnaḥ saṃvāahanāani ça (A. Sam. Sū 5/10)

442. *Imāanṣtu thāarēyēḍdhēgāaṇ hitāarthēe pretya çhēha ça*
Sāahasāanāamaśaṣtāanāaṃ manōvāakkāayakarmaṇāaṃ (Ch. Sū 7/26)

443. *Puṇyaśabdō vipāapaṭwāaṇmanōvāakkāayakarmaṇaaṃ*
Dharmāarthakāamāaṇpuruṣaḥ sukhēe bhuṇkē çhinōti ça (Ch. Sū 7/30)

Important Facts related to Diet

1. Diet

It is a known fact that food is vital for health. It is important to know, not only what to eat, but also when to eat and the qualities of what is consumed. Only then can we enjoy all the benefits that food has to offer us. Some important facts about food are given below:

♦ Unctuous (smooth/oily) Food[444]

Our diet must contain adequate amount of *ghēe* and oil. Fearing heart diseases, blood pressure and obesity, people avoid *ghēe* and other oils which does more harm than good. *Ghēe* and other oils not only enrich the taste, but also soften food and hasten digestion, strengthen the body, sharpen senses, improve complexion, transport *vāyu* and aid in smooth elimination of wastes. They lubricate the joints reducing wear and tear due to friction. Now days popularity of refined oil has increased susceptibility to joint disorders. Hence, it is essential to have ghee, oil and other facts in our diet.

♦ Fresh and Warm Food[445]

Food should always be freshly prepared and eaten warm as it is nourishing, tasty, easy to digest, and regulates *vāyu*. It also boosts digestion. Cold and stale food is *taamsik* and has no nutrition.

♦ Appearance

The colour, aroma and taste of food create a desire to eat and stimulate the digestive juices. Hence, attention must be paid to its appearance and presentation. This is particularly true for patients, as a restricted diet tends to make them disinterested in food.

♦ Place of Eating

The place where food is taken should be clean, pleasant and peaceful. Dirty, noisy or disorganized surroundings disturbs peace of mind, which adversely affects not only the appetite, but also the entire digestive process. Eating food should be treated as a sacred activity and hence must be performed with the same kind of earnestness and concentration. Eating while watching television or talking on the telephone should be avoided.

♦ Mental State

Eating when angry, jealous, tense, nervous, scared etc. prevents one from enjoying food. The secretion of digestive juices is also hampered. Hence, discussing, watching,

---

444. *Ṣnighamaṣ́nēeyāaṭ ṣnēeyāaṭ ṣnigdhaṃ hi bhujyāmāanaṃ ṣwadatē*
bhukṭaṃ ḉhāanudēeṛṇamagnimudēerayati, kṣipraṃ jarāaṃ jarāaṃ gaḉhhati
Vāatamahulōmayati, śarēeramupaḉhinōti, ḍriḍikarōtiṇḍṛiyāaṇi
balāabhiṿriḍdhimupajanayati, varṇaprasāadaṃ chāabhinivaṛtayati (Ch. Vi. 1/24/2)

445. *Uṣ́ṇamanēeyāata uṣ́naṃ hi bhujyamāanaṃ ṣwadatē,*
bhukṭaṇḉhāagnimāudaṛyamudēerayati, kṣipraṃ jarāaṃ gaḉhhati,
Vāatamanulōmayati ṡlēṣmāaṇaṃ ḉha pariḥrāaṣyati,
taṣmāaduṣṇamaṣ́nēeyāata (Ch. Vi. 1/24/11)

reading or thinking about disturbing things while eating should be avoided.

♦ Timings

For smooth and complete digestion, it is of vital importance that food be eaten only at the appropriate and regular hour. A few things must be kept in mind while deciding when to eat. Food should not be consumed in the following circumstances:

- Absence of hunger.
- Before the complete digestion of the last meal. (If food is eaten before the complete digestion of the preceding meal, its undigested *ras* gets mixed with the *ras* of the fresh meal, thus aggravating all the *doshas* and making the body susceptible to a variety of ailments)
- If experiencing eructation from the last meal.
- Feeling heaviness in the heart or stomach.
- Before waste elimination (expulsion of gas, urine and stool).

If food is eaten during the period of *pitta* increase (for eg.between 12 to 2 pm), it gets digested very quickly and maximum nutrition is derived from the food consumed.

It is a common experience that hunger is felt at the regular hours of eating. Something must always be eaten at such times as digestive juices are being secreted, and if nothing is eaten, they aggravate *pitta* causing harm to the body. Weakness, fatigue, body-ache, disinterest in food, change in complexion, weakening of eyesight etc. are felt when eating is avoided even on feeling hungry. If food is eaten after the regular hours, it does not get digested properly, as the body is not ready to absorb food due to the effect of heightened *vāyu* after the passage of mealtime.

♦ Quantity[446]

To obtain maximum nutrition, food should be taken in the appropriate quantity. One third of the stomach must remain empty after eating. This is essential for proper mixing of digestive fluids with food. If the stomach is packed to capacity, digestion is hindered disrupting the entire process of food absorption and assimilation.

If, after a meal, hunger is satisfied, heaviness in the chest region and stomach is absent, and no difficulty in standing, sitting, sleeping,

---

446. *Kuśēraprapēedanamāahāarēṇa, ḥridayaṣyāanavarōdhaḥ, pāarṣvayōra*
-vipāaṭanaṃ, natigāuravamudaraṣya, pṛēeṇanamiṇdriyāaṇāaṃ
Ḳṣuṭpipāasōparamaḥ, ṣthāanaasanaśayanagama nōçhçhhawāasa
Ṛraśwāasahāaṣyasaṇkathāasu sukhāanuvṛittiḥ, sāayaṃ pṛāataṣcha
Sukhēṇ pariṇamaṉaṃ, balavaṛṇnopaçchayakaraṭwaṃ çha iti māatrāavatō
lakṣaṇamāahāaraṣya bhavati (Ch.Vi. 2/6)
Māatrāa punaḥ piṇdapariṇāamataḥ samudāayēna pratiḍravyāapēkṣayāa
çhāahāaraṛāaśiḥ (A.S. Su 10/9)
Ṭrividhaṃ ḳuśāu ṣthāapayēdavakāaśāaṇśamāahāaraṣyāahāaramupayuṇjāanaḥ
taḍyathāa-āikamavakāaśāaṃśaṃ mōoṛtāanāamāahāaravikāarḥāaṃ
āikaṃ ḍravāaṇāaṃ, āikaṃ ṗunaṛvāatapiṭṭaṣlēṣmāaṇaṃ
āitāavatēeṃ ḥyāahāaramāatramupayunjāanō nāamāatrāahāarajaṃ
kiṇchidaśubhaṃ pṛāapṇōti (Ch. Vi. 2/3)

walking, laughing, breathing, talking etc. is experienced, then it can be assumed that food has been eaten in appropriate quantity. Other indicators of consumption of food in the right quantity are complete digestion of food before the next meal, expulsion of wind, and absence of any kind of deformation in the *doshas*, *dhātus* and *malas*.

While deciding the quantity of food to be eaten, *prakṛiti* (nature), digestive capacity,digestive nature of food, etc. should be kept in mind. If a person with strong digestion overeats a little, he will not be affected much, but overeating by someone with a weak digestion will prove very harmful. Similarly, larger quantities of light foods like rice and green gram can be digested easily whereas heavier foods eaten in large portions can lead to indigestion. But eating anything in excess, including light foods should be avoided. Heavier foods like Black gram pulse can be made digestible by adding asafoetida and thyme seeds. In brief, inadequate quantity of food would lead to weakness and dissatisfaction while overeating will lead to aversion to food, heaviness in the stomach and the chest region, obesity, indigestion, etc. Hence food should be taken only when hunger is felt, keeping in mind the digestive capacity and nature of food.

♦ Importance of Chewing

The first step of the digestive process is the softening of food in the mouth by saliva. This becomes possible when food is chewed. The more it is chewed; the food becomes more liquid and easy-to-digest. If large chunks are swallowed, the delicate organs of the alimentary canal have to exert a lot of force in order to breakdown the solid food portions before absorption, thus weakening these organs. Besides it hampers complete assimilation of food resulting in acidity, constipation etc.

♦ Suitability of Diet[447]

Suitability means usefulness. Diet that suits and benefits one person might prove harmful for another. Hence, selection of diet must be done very carefully. It is only through observation, practice and experience that we learn what kind of diet suits us best. Whole

❖ **Body :** Different constitutions demand different diets.

❖ **Region :** Suitability changes with a change in place. For eg. rice is good for people living in the southern part of the country, while wheat is more suitable for those in the northern parts.

❖ **Season :** Diet that is nutritious in one season might not be as wholesome in the preceding or the following seasons. For eg. pungent and rough foods are more beneficial in extreme cold, while cold foods are suitable only in summers.

❖ **Ailments :** Diet must be decided keeping in mind the nature of ailment one is suffering from, because sometimes food that is normally beneficial tend to aggravate and inflame certain diseases. Food chosen according to the nature of the illness helps in quick recovery and regaining of complete health.

some foods give maximum nutritional benefits and unwholesome foods can be harmful. Suitability of food is dependent on the following:[448]

If these rules are adhered to while deciding on a suitable diet, then maximum nourishment can be drawn from every bit that is eaten. All *doshas* and *dhātus* then remain healthy and *malas* (waste products) are eliminated regularly. This constitutes good food habits. Eating should be taken very seriously and a busy schedule must not be allowed to disrupt the diet routine. It is an activity, which should be performed with utmost respect and concentration.

An individual, who has a wholesome and appropriate diet, remains healthy and rarely falls ill. During illness merely controlling and regulating diet ensures speedy recovery and medication may not be required. Contrarily, taking the right medication but neglecting to regulate diet, makes recovery very difficult. In some cases unwholesome diet negates the effect of the medication and renders it ineffective by aggravating the cause. Hence, a combination of the right medication and appropriate diet is a must for overcoming ailments and regaining complete health.

"Vinaapi bheśhjāiṛvyārdhi pāṭhyadev nivaṛtate
Na tu pāṭhya viheenasya bheshjaanaam stairopi"

" In absence of medication, a disease can be cured by taking the right kind of diet, but if the right diet is not maintained, all the medicines in the world will be of no use."

Wholesome Diet[449]

Wholesome (beneficial) diet can be described as one that nourishes all *dhatus* of the body, helps restore balance between them when it is disrupted, does not clog the body channels and leads to satisfaction. In contrast, diet, that blocks body channels, is incapable of maintaining

---

447. *Taṭra sāaṭṃyaṃ nāaṃ sahāatṃanāa bhavatyaḅhyaṣtaṃ tadāuçhiṭyāadu paśeta iṭyēkē Sāaṭṃya viparēetamanupaśyāadasāatṃyaṃ* *(A.Su. 10/27)*

448. *Aṇyē punaḥ p̣rakritivayōdēśāṛtudōṣavyāadhivaśeṇa śāatṃyam bahuvidhamiçḥhaṇti Tē ḥyupaśayamāatramaṇgēekṛiṭya Viparēetaguṇawapyupaçḥāarēeṇa sāaṭṃyamāachakṣatē Tulyaguṃamçhāanupaśayāaḍ asāatmyaṃ* *(A.S.Su. 10/28)*

449. *Paṭthyaṃ pathō5napētaṃ yadyaçḥōktaṃ manasaḥ priyaṃ*
Yaçhchāapriyaṃa pathyaṃ çha niyataṃ taṇna lakṣayēt *(Ch. Sū 25/45)*
Māatrāakāalakṛiyāabhōomidēha dōśaguṇāaṇ taraṃ
P̣rāapaya taṭtaddhi ḍriṣyaṇte tē tē bhāavāaratathaa tathāa *(Ch. Sū 25/46)*
Taṣmāaṭ swabhāavō viṛdiṣṭaṣtathāa māatrāadirāaṣrayaḥ
Tadapēkṣyōbhayaṃ kaṛma p̣rayōjyaṃ sidhimiçhichçḥhiṭaa *(Ch. St. 25/47)*
Āahitāagniḥ sadōo paṭhgāaṇyaṇtaṛgnāu juhōti yoḥ
Divasē divaśē ḅrahṃa jayaṭyatha dadāati cha
Naraṃ niḥṣrēyasē yuḳtaṃ sāaṭṃyajgyaṃ pāanabhōjanē
Bhajaṇtē nāamayāaḥ kēchiḍ bhāavinō5pyaṇtarāaḍritē *(Ch. Su27/46-67)*

balance between *dhātus*, causes harm and is disliked, is an unwholesome diet.

Wholesome and unwholesome diet varies from person to person. Wholesome for one might be unwholesome for another. The suitability of diet for a person is governed by age, body consitution, nature, quantity of *dravya* and compatibility with other *dravyas*. Keeping the above in mind one should exclude unwholesome items from ones diet and eat only wholesome foods.

Some foods/substances are by nature wholsesome or unwholesome. They are listed below:

Category	Wholesome	Unwholesome
1. Cereals/ grains with hard seed coat	Red shali rice	Barley Plant *(Yawak)*
2. Pulses	Green gram	Black gram (*uṛad*)
3. Potable waters	Rain water collected before it reaches the ground	River water in rainy season
4. Salt	Rock Salt	Fertile *(Ushar)*
5. Leafy vegetables	*Leptadenia reticulate (Jēevanti leaf)*	Mustard leaf
6. *Ghēe*	Cow milk	Sheep milk
7. Milk	Cow milk	Sheep milk
8. Tubers and Rhizome	Ginger	Potato or jagery
9. Fruit	Grapes	*Khhitij , Lakneh (Barhal))*
10. Products of Sugarcane	Sugar	Phaneet
11. Vegetable oil	*Sesame* oil	Kusum oil *(Safron Flower)*

If the wholesome foods are not eaten properly according to body constitution, season, quantity, age, etc. they can cause harm. Food builds the body. Hence it must be consumed sensibly. Greed and ignorance must not be allowed to dictate diet as it can only lead to disorders and imbalance and cause ailments.

Chapter 6

Anupāan
(Liquids taken after meal and medication) and Characteristics Of Important Liquids

Anupāan is considered very important in *Ayuṛved*[450]. *Anupāan* means liquids that should be taken after meals and medication. *Anupāan* boosts taste. The right kind of liquids lend energy and increase virility. They also create freshness, joy and softness. Appropriate liquids not only calm all *doshas*, but also prevent their accumulation in all *dhātus*[451].

The most important drinks used as *anupāan* are[452] – water, hot and cold water, soup, fruit juice, fermented drinks made from grains, milk, extracts of fruits and herbs. *Anupāan* must be chosen according to its qualities, constitution, *dosha* pattern and the state of illness of the patient and age. It should be taken only in right quantity to ensure quick and easy digestion. Taking more than necessary leads to heaviness and *dosha* aggravation; not taking any causes problems as food fails to gain the softness/consistency required for smooth digestion thus leading to various ailments[453]. Under some conditions, even normal intake of *anupāan* must be avoided, for eg. cough, asthma, injury on chest, excessive saliva secretion, head and neck ailments, sore throat etc.

Ayuṛved recommends *anupāan* according to foods and illness. A brief list is as under:[454]

---

450. *Anu paśçhaaṭ saha vāa pēeyatē iṭyanupāaṇaṃ*
Alpadōśamadōśa vāa5pyanupāanēna jēeṛyati (*A. hri Su. 8/50*)

451. *Anupāanaṃ hitaṃ yukṭaṃ taṛpayaṭyāaś umāanavaṃ*
Sukhaṃ paçhati chāahāaramāayuṣē ҫha balāaya ҫha (*Ch. Su 27/326*)
Anupāanaṃ karoṭōorjāaṃ ṭripti yāaptiṃ ḍraḍāangatāaṃ
Aṇnasanghāataśāithilyā uikḷi iṭtijaṛṇāani ҫha (*A Hri Su*)

452. *Anupāanaṃ himaṃ vāari yavagōdhōomayōṛhitaṃ*
Daḍhni maḍē viṣē ķśāuḍrē kōśṇaṃ piśṭamayēṣu tu (*A. h. Su 8/47-49*)
Śāakamuḍgāa diviķritāu maṣṭutaķrāaṃlakāanjekaṃ
Surāa ķriśāanāaṃ puśṭhyaṛthaṃ ṣthōolāanāaṃ tu madhōodakaṃ

453. *Vaṛjyaṃ tōoṛḍhvajaṭrugadaśvāasakāasapṛasēka hiḍhmāaṣwarabhēdoraḥ*
Ķṣatibhiṛgēetabhāaśyaprasaķṭāiśҫha (*A.S.Sū 10/55*)

454. *Ṣnigdhōśṇaṃ māarutē śaṣtaṃ piṭṭē madhuraśēetalaṃ*
kaphē5nupāanaṃ rōoķśō5śṇaṃ ķṣayē māaṃsarasaḥ paraṃ (*Ch. Sū 27/321*)

Ailment/ Food	*Anupāan*
Kapha vitiation	Hot and dry/harsh
Vāyu vitiation	Hot and smooth (unctuous)
Piṭta vitiation	Sweet and cool
Fasting, physical labour, fatigue and weakness due to excessive walking, talking and sexual activity	Milk
Weakness due to alcohol	Honey in water
Insomnia, obesity, fatigue, giddiness, emaciation, cool, heavy, excessive and inappropriate meals	Milk
Bleeding	Milk/sugarcane juice
Poisoning	Salted water prepared with *harad* (myrobalan)
With oily substances	Warm water
(*Bhilawa*) oil	Cold water
(*Shaali*) rice, green gram and foods containing these	Milk
Black gram pulse (black gram) *Pithi* and *pithhi* preparations	Curd, curd water, fermented drinks Oil, soup and fermented drinks
Honey	Water
Curd, pudding, (pasti etc.)	Cold or normal water

Water is the primary *anupaan*, being the most often used, and the most easily available[455].

1. Water

Pure water is like nectar. It is the life-giving liquid whose absence results in death. Clean and normal water cures *piṭta* and toxic accumulation, relieves giddiness, irritation, indigestion, fatigue, dizziness, intoxication and vomiting, and strengthens the heart. Water changes its properties on being boiled, boiled and cooled, warmed and cooled. These properties must be kept in mind while using water[456].

---

455. *Anupāanaṃ tu salilamēva ś̤rēṣ̤thaṃ*
Saṛvarasayōniṭwāaṭsaṛvabhōotasāaṭṃyaṭṃyaṭwāajjēevanāadignṇayōgāachç̣ha (*A.S. Sū 10/42*)

♦ **Pure and drinkable water:**[457]

Rainwater that has not touched the ground is pure because on reaching the earth's surface, the conditions on the ground affect it. Collecting rainwater for individual use is a tedious and almost impossible job. Hence, tap water can be used after it has been boiled and cooled. Boiling purifies water as it then becomes a good medium for digestion and acquires ability to calm vitiated *doshas*.

♦ **Time, quantity and process of water intake**

Time, quantity and process of water intake are very crucial. Excessive water weakens digestion. On the other hand, drinking very little or no water at all obstructs digestion. It also leads to contracting various illnesses, as enough urine and stool is not produced causing accumulation of toxic wastes in the body. Drinking a little water at frequent intervals rather than a lot at one go, is recommended. This not only fulfills the water requirement of the body, it also boosts digestion. Water acts as a medicine during indigestion. Drinking water after food is digested, lends strength to the body.

Drinking water before eating weakens digestion and leads to loss of weight. Water intake during a meal boosts digestion and increases life-span. Water taken an hour after a meal, strengthens the body and increases body mass. One must avoid drinking water before a meal. Plump and fat people should drink water during a meal, and thin people, after the meal. Water intake after a meal is harmful for overweight and physically strong people[458].

Although water intake is beneficial for everyone at all times, under some conditions like anorexia, cold with a long history, excessive salivation, oedema, emaciation, weak digestion, obstinate abdominal ailment, skin diseases like leprosy, eye ailments, injury and diabetes its quantity should be reduced[459]. But one must be cautious as not drinking water at all also leads to various disorders. The state and quantity of water should be determined by the circumstances, only then is it fully nourishing. Cold water is useful to people suffering from indigestion and burning sensation in the stomach because it soothes and strengthens digestion, it is

---

456. *Jēevanaṃ tarpaṇaṃ hṛidyaṃ hḷāadi buḍdhi prabodhaṇaṃ*
Taṇva ṿgakṭarasaṃ ṃriṣṭaṃ śēetaṃ śuçhyaṃritōpamaṃ (A.S.Su. 6/3)

457. *Khāatapataṭ sōmavāayṿarkāiḥ ṣpriṣṭaṃ kāalāanuvaṛtibhiḥ*
Śēetōṣṇaṣnigdharōokṣāadhāiṛythāasaṇnaṃ mahēeguṇāiḥ (Ch. Sū 27/197)

458. *Bhakṭaṣyāadāu jalaṃ pēetamagnisāadaṃ kṛiśāaṇgaṭāaṃ* (AS.Sū 6/41)
Aṇtē karōti ṣthōolaṭwamōoṛdhvaṃ çhāamāaśayāaṭ kaphaṃ
Maḍhyē maḍhyāaṇgatāaṃ sāaṃyaṃ dhāatōonāaṃ jaraṇaṃ sukhaṃ (A.S. Sū 6/42)

459. *Anavaṣthitadōśāagnēṛvyāadhi kśēeṇabalaṣya cha*
Nāalṗamapỵāamamudakaṃ hitaṃ taḍdhi ṭridōśakṛiṭ (A.S.Su 6/38)
Tējasaḥ ṗratipakśaṭwāaṇmaṇdāaghiṛvaṛjayējjalaṃ
Saṛvameva tathāa ṣyaṇdaṗlēehāaviḍradhigulṃinaḥ (Sū 6/39)
Pāaṇdōodarāatisāarāa śograhaṇēeśoṣaśophinaḥ
Kāamamalṗamaśakṭāu tu pēyamāuṣadhasaṇṣkritaṃ (Su 6/40)

harmful for people suffering from asthma, cold etc. Therefore, it becomes necessary to understand the qualities and effects of different types of water.

♦ Conditions in which water intake after food should be avoided

People who suffer from diseases caused due to *vāyu* aggravation like hiccups, asthma, cough, tuberculosis, head ailments etc should not take water after meals and people who have to sing or speak loudly, should not drink water after meals. During head ailments, water does not go downwards which causes the *vāyu* to be further aggravated. Normally the oily parts of the meal calm the *vāyu*, but water, which is cold, aggravates it.

People, who have to strain their vocal cords more than usual, should avoid after-meal water intake as it washes down the essential oils taken in with the meal. These oils are important as they are soothing. On their removal, the throat becomes dry leading to throat disorders. Some experts feel that water intake obstructs assimilation of nutrients during digestion leading to ailments.

♦ Cold Water[460]

Cold water is curative during a fainting fit, burning sensation caused by aggravated *pitta*, blood vitiation, intoxication, dizziness, vomiting, fatigue, dyspnoea *(tamak shwas)* and bleeding. It is also digestion boosting.

However, cold water is harmful in the following conditions

Pain in the ribs, cold, sore throat, distension, cataract, anorexia, sprue syndrome, asthma, cough, hiccups, boils, and after eating oily food[461].

♦ Hot Water[462]

Hot water is light. It strengthens digestion and cures digestive disorders. It also cures chronic cold, distension, hiccups, and effects of aggravated *vayu* and water.

Boiled water is pure. When it is boiled till only three fourths of the original quantity is left, it acquires properties to cure *vāyu* and *vāyu* engendered diseases. When only half of it is left, it is called *usna* (talicire) water and cures *tridoshas* (*vāyu*, *pitta* and *kapha*) and diseases related to them. It purifies urine, and benefits people suffering from asthma,

---

460. *Śēetaṃ madāaṭyayaglāanimōorçhhāarḍiśramabḥramāaṇ*
Ṭriśṇōṣmadāahapiṭṭāaṣrigviṣaṇyaṃbu çha nihaṇti taṭ **(A. S. Sū 6/43)**
(Su Su 45/29)

461. *Pāarṣvaśōolē pratiśyaayē vāataroḡē galagrahē*
Āaḍhmāanē ṣtimitē kōṣthē saḍyaḥ śuḍḍhē navajwarē
Hikkāayāaṃ ṣnēhapēetē çha śēetāaṃbu parivarjayēṭ **(Su. Sū 45/30)**

462. *Kaphamedō5nilamaghnaṃ dēepaṇaṃ baṣtiśoḍhanaṃ*
śwāasakāasajwaraharaṃ pathyamuśṇōdakaṃ sadāa **(Su Sū 45/39)**
Kśēeṇa pāadaṭrabhāagāarḍhaṃ dēśarṭugurulāaghavāaṭ
Kwathitaṃfēnarahitaṃ vēgamamalaṃ hitaṃ
Hi ḍhmāa55ḍhmāanāanilaśmaṭriṭkāasaśwāaspēenasē
Pāarṛṣva śōolāamamēdaḥsu saḍyaḥ śuḍḥāu navajwarē
Dēepanaṃ pāachananḳaṇṭhyaṃ laghu vaṣṭiviśōdhanaṃ **(A. S. Sū 6/44-55)**

cough, fever and digestive problems. Drinking hot water at night dissolves accumulated *kapha*, and eliminates wind and stool.

When only one fourth of the original quantity is left, it is called *ārogyāṃbu*. It is nourishing, light and digestive, and strengthens digestive fire *(jathrāgni)*. Warm *ārogyāṃbu* is very light and it relieves asthma, cough, aggravated *kapha*, constipation, distension in stomach, anaemia, shooting pains, piles, pseudo tumour, fever, oedema, and stomach ache. It also relieves rib pain, severe stomach ache and hiccups, excessive thirst, *shool*, vomiting, diarrhoea, *vāyu* and *kapha* digestion. It also purifies urine[463].

When water is boiled and then cooled it is called *shritsheet*. It is very good for people suffering from burning sensation, diarrhoea, fainting, intoxication, poisoning, nausea, dizziness, excessive thirst, vitiated *piṭta* and blood, disorders caused by *kapha* and *piṭta* and alcoholic substances and simultaneous aggravation of all three *doshas*.

If after boiling, water is cooled in the same container which is kept covered, it becomes very light. It does not block *srotas* and cures aggravation of all three *doshas*, worms in the stomach, excessive thirst and fever.

If water is transferred to another container before cooling, it is called *dhārāśheet*. It is heavy as it contains air. This water requires time for absorption and can cause constipation.

Boiled water becomes heavy after 24 hours and is not easily absorbed. It also aggravates all three *doshas*[464].

♦ *Haṇsodak* Or *Aṇshudak* Water (Water Kept In Sunlight And Moonlight):[465]

Water kept in the sunlight during the day is called *'haṇsodak'* and kept in the moon light at night is called *'aṇshudak'*

463. *Maḍyapāanāatṣamuḍbhōotē rōgē piṭtōṭhitē tathāa*
Saṇnipāatasamuṭwē ċha śritaśēetaṃ praśaṣyatē (42)
Dāahāatisāara pittāasringnōorċhhāamadyavisartiṣu
Śritaśēetaṃ jalaṃ śaṣtaṃ trisṇāaċhċhhardiḅhramēṣu ċha (Su. Sū 45/43)

464. *Tōyaṃ vaṇhiguṇaḅhraṣṭaṃ pāakē5mlaṃ saṛvadōśaṛkriṭ* (A.S. Sū 6/48)
Bhaveṭ paṛyuṣitaṃ taċhcha
Na ċha paṛyaṣitaṃ dēyaṃ kadāachidvāari jāanatāa
Aṃlēebhōotaṃ kaphōṭklēśi na vitaṃ taṭ pipāasavē (Su. Sū 45/41)

465. *Divāa sōoṛyāaṇśu saṇtriptaniśiċhaṇdrāaṇśuśēetalam*
Kāalēna pakvaṃ niṛdōśaṃagaṣyēnāaviṣiḳritaṃ
Haṇsōdakaṃ iti ḳhyāataṃ śāaradaṃ vinalaṃ śuchi
ṣṇāana pāanāanavagāahēṣu śaṣyatē taḍyathāa5ṃritam (Ch. Su 6/46-47)
Divāadivāakarakorāiṛniśāakarkarāiṛnisi
Saṇtaptaṃ ḥlāaditaṃ tōyamagaṣṭyēnāaviṣēekṛitaṃ (A.S.Sū 4/56)
Nōṛḍhwāaṇgamāarutāaviṣṭāa na hikḳāaśwāaṣakāasinaḥ
Na gēetabhāa ṣyāaḍhyayanaprasaḳtāa nōrasi ḳṣatāaḥ
Pibēyurudakaṃ bhuḳṭwāa taḍdhi kaṇthōrasi ṣthitaṃ
Ṣnēhamāahāarajaṃ hatwāa bhōoyō dōṣaaya kalpatē (Charak Sutra 27/327-328)

This water is considered to be similar to nectar. It is unctuous and has a calming effect on all three *doshas*. It is cool and digestive, boosts energy and intelligence, slows the onslaught of old age ailments, and does not obstruct the flow of body fluids in *srotas*. It is free from all the doshas

♦ Water Intake In The Morning

If water is taken first thing in the morning before eating or drinking anything else, it prevents wrinkles, grey hair, hoarse throat, aggravated cold, asthma, constipation and tuberculosis.

♦ Water According To Seasons

Summer and winter *(shisir):* water boiled to 1/4th its original quantity

Winter, rains and spring :water boiled in ìts original quantity

♦ Time Required For Absorption

Water that is not boiled takes 3 hours, boiled and cooled takes 1.5 hours and boiled water that is drunk warm takes 45 minutes to be absorbed. It is clear that while the first type is the heaviest, the third is the lightest. One must choose water according to one's digestive capacity.

♦ Identifying Impure Water[466]

The easily identifiable impure water is the one that contains foreign bodies like mud, leaves, mosquitoes, etc. Water that smells or has changed colour is also impure. Water that has no access to sunlight and moonlight is also considered unfit for consumption. Water from unexpected rains, or water collected from the ground immediately after rains is impure. One should not only avoid drinking it, but also refrain from bathing in it.

Water and its impurities are as follows:

1. ***Sparsh* impurity:** Water that is rough, harsh and sticky to touch.
2. ***Rōop* impurity:** Water containing foreign bodies like leaves, dust etc. and one that has changed colour.
3. ***Ras* impurity:** Water with distinct taste. Eg. Saline water.
4. ***Gandh* impurity:** Water that has odour.
5. ***Virya* impurity:** Water which takes time to be absorbed, induces thirst or salivation, and causes heaviness.

Consuming water with these impurities can lead to external (boils, pimples, itching, dry skin and other skin related problems) and internal (disorders of digestion,constipation,

---

466. *Kēeṭāahimōotṛaviṭkōthaṭriṇajāalōṭkaṭāavilaṃ*
Paṇkapaṇkajaśāivāalahathaṛnāadisaṇṣṭritaṃ

Sōoṛyēṇdu pavanāaḍri ṣṭaṃ ju ṣṭaṃ ḉha kṣ̌uḍrajaṇtubhiḥ
Abhivṛiṣ̌ṭaṃ vivaṛnaṃ ḉha kaluṣaṃ ṣṭhōolafēnilaṃ

Virasaṃ gaṇdhavaṭ taptaṃ daṇtagrāahyatiśāiṭyataḥ
Anāarṭavaṃ ḉha yadiḍvyamāarṭavaṃ prathamaṃ ḉha yaṭ

Lōotāaditaṇtuviṇmōotṛaviṣasaṇṣ̌lēṣadōoṣitaṃ
Tatkuṛyāaṭ ṣnāana pāanāabḥyāaṃ triṣ̌ṇāaśsḍhmāanōdarajwaraaṇ

Kāa sāagnisāadāabhi ṣyaṇda kaṇdōogaṇdāadikāaṇataḥ
Talyarjayēdabhāavē vāa tōyaṣyāaṇyaṣya śaṣyatē *(AS. Sū 6/21-25)*

loose motions, vomiting, etc.) disorders.

If clean water is not available, and one is forced to use impure water, it is a must that the water be purified before consumption. These are several ways of doing so - exposing it to sunlight, cooling a burning lump of gold, silver, stone, sand or mud in impure water seven times, straining water through a clean piece of cloth or using a filter[467].

Some Other Useful Substances

There are several food items that we use frequently in total ignorance of their qualities, effects and benefits. Let's learn about a few in the following pages and get to know their qualities. This will help us to choose only those substances that suit us and direct us how to change the potentially harmful substances to suit our body constitution.

2. Coconut Water[468]

Coconut water that is naturally available is smooth, sweet, nourishing, cool, strengthening and easily digestible. It relieves excessive thirst, *piṭta*, *vāyu* and heat in the liver, increases digestive ability and cleans the urinary organs. Therefore, drinking coconut water in all seasons especially in summers is health enhancing. Artificial aerated drinks can be replaced by this naturally occurring nourishing drink.

Together with water, other liquids like milk, *ghēe*, oil etc. are used regularly. Not being aware of their properties and effects can lead to their misuse. Hence, here is a brief description of each.

3. Milk[469]

Milk is believed to be nectar. The taste essence of milk is sweet (except camel milk which is salty), *vipak* is sweet, oily, heavy, *virya* is cool. It calms *piṭta* and *vāyu* and increases *kapha.* It improves intelligence, provides strength and nourishment and builds *dhātus*. Because it has all the qualities of *ojas*, milk replenishes it. Milk also adds to the life energy, relieves constipation, stops bleeding, lends unctuousness to the body, helps in conception, aids healing of wounds, improves complexion, strengthens voice and relieves burning and irritation. It is also beneficial during tuberculosis, chronic fever, and hyper acidity, stomach-ache after meals, stomach disorders, constipation, low semen, and emaciation. It also guards against old age deformities. Regular intake of milk and *ghēe*

467. *Pāaṣāaṇarōopyaṃriḍdhēmaja tutāapāaṛkatāapitaṃ*
Pāanēeyamuśṇaṃ śēetaṃ vāa tridōśaghnaṃ triḍṛtjiṭ
Laghvarōokṣaṃ ḳlamaghnaṃ cha toyaṃ ḳwathita śēetalaṃ
Saṇsaṛgē piṭṭakaphayōḥ saṇnipāatē ḉha śaṣyatē

468. *Nāarikēlōdakaṃ ṣnigdhaṃ ṣwāadu ṿriśyaṃ hiananḷaghu*
Ṭriśṇāapiṭṭāanilaharaṃ dēepanaṃ baṣtiśodhanaṃ
ṣnigdhaṃ ṣwāadu himaṃ hridyaṃ dēepaṇaṃ baṣtiśodhanaṃ **(A. Sa. Sū. 6/51)**
Ṿri ṣyaṃ piṭtapipāasāaghnaṃ nāarikēlōdakaṃ guru **(Su. Sū 45/44)**

is nourishing. Cow milk is considered the best and sheep milk the least nourishing.

♦ Cow Milk[470]

Cow milk is sweet, unctuous, heavy, cool, nourishing, boosts strength, intelligence and milk formation, strengthens life force, does not accumulate in *srotas*, and very beneficial for people recovering from sickness or injury. It is also very useful for people suffering from dizziness due to fatigue, intoxication, excessive thirst, *vāas*, cough, old fever, problems with urine elimination, and bleeding. It calms *vata* and *piṭta doshas*. Milk from a cow varies with the difference in the colour of the cowhide and in the uterus. The milk from a young cow is sweet, nourishing and calming all three *doshas*. Milk from an old cow is not as nourishing. Similarly, milk from black cow calms *vāyu dosha* and is better in quality than milk from a yellow/white cow, which calms both *vāyu* and *pitta doshas*.

♦ Buffalo Milk[471]

Buffalo milk is cooler, heavier and more unctuous than cow milk. It also accumulates in the *srotas* more than cow milk. It is very good for people with sharp or corrosive digestive power, and people suffering from insomnia. It is considered one of the best sedatives. Although the quality of *ghēe* from

---

469. *Madhuraṃ piçhhilaṃ śēetaṃ ṣnigdhaṃ ślakṣ̄naṃ saraṃmridu*
Sar̄vaprāaṇabhritāaṃ taṣmāaṭ sāaṭmyaṃ kṣēeramihōçhyatē (Su. Sū 45/48)
Prāayaśō madhuraṃ ṣnigdhaṃ śēetaṃ ṣtanyaṇ payō mataṃ
Prēeṇanaṃ ḅrinhaṇaṃ ṿri ṣyaṃ madhyaṃ balyaṇmanaṣkaraṃ
Jēevanēeyaṃ ṣramaharaṃ śwāasakāasanibaṛhaṇaṃ
Haṇti śōṇita pittaṃ çha sahdhāanaṃ vihataṣya çha
Saṛvaprāaṇabhlitāaṃ sāaṭmyaṃ śamanaṃ śodhanaṃ tathāa
Ṭriśṇāaghaaṃ dēepaēeyaṇçha ṣrē ṣthaṃ ḳ sēeṇaḳ satēṣu çha
Pāaṇdurōgē5ṃlapiṭtē çha śōṣē gulmē tathōdarē
Atēesāarē jwarē dāahē ṣwayathāu cha vi ṣēṣataḥ
Yōniśuḳra dōśēṣu mōotrēṣu pradarēṣu çha
Purēesē grathitē pathyaṃ vāatapiṭtavikāariṇāaṃ
Naṣyāalepāavagāahēṣu vamanāaṣthāapanēṣu cha
Virēçhanē ṣnēhanē çha payaḥ saṛvaṭra yujyatē (Ch. Sū 1/108-112)

470. *Aṭra gaṿyaṃ tu jēevanēeyaṃ rasāayanaṃ* (A.Sā.Sū 6/54-55)
Ḳsata ḳṣēeṇahitaṃ medhyaṃ vaṛnyaṃ ṣtanyakaraṃ saraṃ
Śramaḅhramamadāalaśṃēeśwāasakāasāatiṭriṭḳṣudhaḥ
Jēeṛna jwaraṃ mōotraḳriçhehḥraṃ raḳtapiṭtaṃ çha nāaśayēṭ
Ṣwāadu śēetaṃ ṃridu ṣnigdhaṃ bahalaṃ ślaḳṣ̄napiçhçhhilaṃ
Guru maṇdaṃ prasaṇnaṃ çha gaṿyaṃ daśaguṇaṃ payaḥ
Tadēvaṇguṇamēvāujaḥ sāamāaṇyāadabhivaṛdhayēṭ
Ṗravara jēevanēeyāanāaṃ ḳṣēeramaḳtaṃ rasāayanaṃ (Ch. Sū 27/217-218)

471. *Mahiṣēeṇāaṃ gurutaraṃ gaṿyāaçhçhhēetataraṃ puyaḥ*
Ṣnēhāaṇyōonamaniḍrāaya hitamaṭyagnayē çha taṭ (Ch. Sū 27/219)
Hitamatyagṇyaniḍrēḅhyō garēeyō māahisaṃ himaṃ (A.S.Sū 6/56)

cow milk is said to be better, buffalo milk contains a larger quantity.

♦ Goat Milk[472]

Goat milk is not as widely used as cow and buffalo milk. It is sweet and has a pungent/astringent flavour to it. It is cool and easily digestible. Goat milk has medicinal properties. Patients of diarrhoea, TB, fever, asthma, bleeding, cough and poisoning benefit from drinking goat milk. It also boosts digestion.

Milk boiled without adding water is heavy and oily. If water is added and it is boiled till the water evaporates, it becomes light. Adding long pepper, dry ginger, turmeric and liquorice reduces its *kapha* aggravating properties.

Unheated milk has a tendency to accumulate in the *srotas* and is heavy, while heated milk is light and does not accumulate in the *srotas*. It is best to drink cow milk that has been boiled, buffalo milk that has been cooled after milking, and goat milk that has been cooled after boiling.

Milk extracted in the morning is heavier and cooler than milk collected in the evening. Milk must be taken at night to calm the irritation caused by food intake during the daytime. It is said that a man who begins the day with a glass of water, has diluted curd after lunch, and drinks a glass of milk before going to sleep, remains ever healthy and free of illness.

If the taste, colour and smell of milk is found altered, it should not be drunk. Salty and sour things should not be taken with milk. These combinations can lead to diseases like leprosy. Milk-cream is oil-rich, calms *vāyu* and *piṭta* and increases semen. Milk of a cow that has been recently calved, is heavy, accumulating (thick), *kapha* strengthening and protein-rich. *Khoyā* (thickened milk) is heavy, oily, strengthening and semen boosting. Cottage cheese and curdled milk is also strength providing but is lighter than *khoya*. Water left after curdling milk is also very good. A glass of this water contains 50 calories. It is very beneficial for people suffering from weak digestion.

4. Curd[473]

Curd is heavy, oily, accumulating, and sour in taste essence and after taste, cures wind and constipation, increases *kapha*, *piṭta*, blood, physical strength, semen and digestive power. It is nourishing and boosts appetite. It is beneficial for people suffering from stomach disorders, cold and inflammation of nose, malaria, emaciation, and fever due to cold and urinary disorders, especially urine elimination. Excessive and improper consumption of curd can cause swelling, blood ailments, fever, bleeding and jaundice.

---

472. *Alpāaṃbupāana vyāayāamakaṭutikṭāaśanāirlaghu*
Aajaṃ śōṣajwara śwāasaraḳtapiṭṭāatisāarajit *(A.S. Sū - 6/57)*
Çhhāagaṃ kaṣāayamadhuraṃ śēetaṃ grāahi payō laghu
Raḳtapiṭṭaatisāaraghnaṃ ḳśayakāasajwarāapahaṃ *(Ch. Sū 27/222)*

♦ **Curd cream :** provides strength, increases semen, and is beneficial during blood piles.

♦ **Curd water :**[474] light, increases digestion, cleans *srotas*, regulates wind and other waste products.

♦ **Butterless curd:** rough, wind producing, increases wind and constipation, but beneficial for colitis disorders.

♦ **Unset curd:** this is curd that is not ready and should not be used.

♦ **Procedure for usage**[475]

Curd should not be eaten at night. Curd should not be eaten without one of the following – *ghēe*, honey, sugar, green gram or gooseberry. It should not be warmed or heated. and used in summer, spring and winter seasons. Rains and mild winters are suitable seasons for curd consumption.

5. Buttermilk[476]

Buttermilk is prepared by adding water to curd or churning it without water. Depending on the kind of curd used, buttermilk can be sweet or sour. The qualities of buttermilk varies according to the quantity of water and oil butter in it. Buttermilk made by churning curd without adding water is called *Ghol*, that which has one fourth water is *takr*, when the quantity of water is fifty percent it is called *uḍśhwit*. Buttermilk that has no butter in it is called '*mathit*'. When adequate amount of water is added to '*mathit*', it is called *chhach*.

---

473. *Rōchanaṃ dēepanaṃ vriśyaṃ ṣhēhanaṃ balavardhanaṃ*
Pāakē5ṃlamuśṇaṃ vāataghnaṃ maṇgalyaṃ brihanaṃ dadhi
Pēenasē chāatisāarē ċha śeetakē viṣanajwarē
Aruchāu mōoṭrakṛiċhċhharē ċha kāarśyē ċha dadhi śaṣyatē (*Charak Sū 27/225-226*)
Alpapāakarasaṃ grāahi gurōosṇaṃ dadhi vāatajiṭ
Mēdaḥ śukrabalaślēṣmarakṭapiṭṭāagniśōphakṛiṭ
Rōchiśṇu śaśtamaruchāu śēetakē viṣamājwarē
Pēenasē mōotrakṛiċhċharē ċha rōokṣaṃ tu granēegadē (*AS. Sū 6/65-66*)

474. *Tavaṇmaṣtu saraṃ ṣrōtaḥśōdhi vi ṣṭaṃbhajiḷḷaghu* (*ASSū 6/71*)

475. *Nāivāadyāaṇniśinaivōśṇaṃ vasantōśṇaśaraṭsu na*
Nāamuga5ōopaṃ nāaśaudraṃ tatrāaḍhritasitōpalaṃ
Na chāanāamalakaṃ nāapi niṭyaṃ nō maṇdamaṇyathāa
Jwarāaṣrikapiṭṭavēesairpakuśtha pāaṇḍubhrama pradaṃ (*A.S. Sū 6/67-68*)
Na naḳtaṃ dadhi bhuṇjeeṭ na chāapya ghritaśaṛkaraṃ
Nāamuḍgayōosaṃ nāakśaudraw nōsṇaṃ nāamalakaiṛvināa
Jwarāaṣrikpiṭṭavēesaṛpaku ṣtha pāaṇḍvyaḅhramāaṇ
Ṗrāapnuyāaṭ kāamalāaṃ chōgrāaṃ vidhiṃ hiṭwāa dadhipriyaḥ (*Ch. Sū 7/61-62*)

476. *Maṇthanāadi ṗrithagbhōotaṣnēhamaḍḍhōdakaṃ ċha yaṭ*
Nāatisāaṇḍraḍraḍravaṃ takraṃ swāaḍvaṃlaṃ tuvaraṃ rasē (*Su. Sū 45/85*)

Their qualities are as follows:

Ghol	calms *vāyu* and *piṭta doshas*
Takr	calms all three *doshas*
Uḍśhwit	increases *kapha*
Mathit	*kapha* and *piṭta* shaamak *(calming)*
Chhach	light, cool, calming *vāat* and *piṭta*, increases *kapha*. Taken with salt it increases digestion. *Takr* with no butter content is very light. Buttermilk that is made without extracting any butter content is heavy, strengthening and *kapha* boosting.

General qualities of buttermilk[477]

Takr is light, sweet, astringent, sweet in after taste, *kapha-vāat* calming, increases digestion, *srota* purifying, causing constipation, good for heart, urine increasing. It is beneficial for people suffering from piles, swelling, stomach disorders, urine elimination problems, and spleen, and gum disorders caused due to *ghēe*, poisoning and jaundice. Modern science has also confirmed that buttermilk is good for people suffering from calorie related heart problems.

Fresh buttermilk destroys *kapha* from abdominal organs, and enhances *piṭta*. Patients with inflammation of the nose, cough, asthma and throat problems should use matured buttermilk.

Buttermilk is the most potent remedy for *kapha* and *vāyu* disorders. Its effectiveness changes with the condiments added to it:

Sour buttermilk+dried ginger and rock salt	cures *vāyu* disorders
Sweet buttermilk+sugar	cures *piṭta* disorders
Buttermilk+*trikuti* (dry ginger+ black pepper+ Long pepper) and salt of barley (yavkshaar)	cures *kapha* disorders
Buttermilk+asfoetida+cumin seeds	destroys *vāyu* and piles, diarrhoea, pain in the genital region, increases digestion
Buttermilk+jaggery	cures urination disorders-
Buttermilk+Leadwort *(chiṭrak)*	cures jaundice disorders

477. *Taķraṃ laghu kaṣāayāaṃlaṃ dēepanaṃ kaphavāatajiṭ*
śōphō darāaṛśograhaṇēedōoṣamōotragrahāaruchēeḥ
Gulmaplēehāaghritvyāapadgarapāanḍvāamayāaṇ jayēṭ. *(A.S. Sū 6/69-70)*

Sour buttermilk is harmful. Buttermilk of any kind should be avoided when suffering from injury on chest, emaciation, giddiness, fainting, irritation and bleeding. It should also be avoided during summer[478].

6. Butter[479]

There are two types of butter: (i) made from curd: it is sweet, astringent, and has sweet *vipak.* It is light, oily, *shēetvirya*, calms *vāyu-piṭta*, promotes *varn agni*, assimilating, boosts digestion, increases semen, intelligence and lends strength to the heart. It is beneficial for people suffering from anorexia, cough, piles, and paralysis. (ii) Made from milk: this is very cool, beneficial for eyes, assimilation and counters bleeding. It is an excellent medicine for people suffering from paralysis[480].

7. *Ghēe* (Clarified Butter)

Ghēe is the best among all oily substances due to unique quality of increasing the potency of herbal preparations. *Ghēe* made from cow milk is considered the most superior among all varieties of *ghēe*.

Ghēe is heavy, oily, has sweet after taste, *shēetvirya*, and enhances intelligence, strength, life span, semen, vision, fertility, glow, tenderness and sound quality. It is nourishing and lends stability to the body. It fortifies the heart and provides nourishment even during old age. Its medicinal and nourishing properties make it useful for people suffering from mental disturbances, fever, irritation and inflammation, stress, emaciation, anorexia, injury and burning. It regulates *vāyu* and boosts digestive powers. It flushes out *doshas* from *srotas*, clearing and lubricating them[481].

Ghēe is used in diverse ways: as a part of diet, with medicinal preparations, for massage, enema, and *nasya* treatments (inhalation).

Inhalation during bleeding, massage with matured *ghēe* during *pāarśhvshōol*, and as a part of diet during mental disturbances, weakness, cough, abortion, chronic fever, and cataract, is recommended. Regular

---

478. *Nāiva takṛaṃ kśate dadẏāaṇnō ṣṇakāalē na duṛbalē*
Na mōorçhhāa ḅhraṃdāahēṣu na rōgē raḳtapaittikē *(ASSu 6/70)*

479. *Śēetaṃ ṣwāadu kaṣāayāaṃlaṃ nanēetaṃ navōḍdhritaṃ*
Yakṣamāa5ṛsōrditapittāa ṣrigvāatajiḍ grāahi dēepanaṃ
Ḳṣēerōḍḅhvaṃ tu saṇgrāahi raḳtapittāaḳsirōgajit *(A.S.Su 6/72)*

480. *Śnēhāaṇāamuṭṭamaṃ śēetaṃ vayasaḥ ṣthāapanaṃ ghritaṃ* *(AS.Sū 6/75)*
Saṛvaṣnēhōṭtamaṃ śēetaṃ madhuraṃ rasapāakayōḥ
Sahaṣravēeṛyaṃ vidhibhirghritaṃ kaṛansahasrakṛit *(Ch. Sū 27/232)*

481. *Śaṣtaṃ dhēesṃritimēdhāagnibilāayuḥ śuḳraçhaḳsuṣāaṃ*
Bāalaṿriḍḍhpṛajāakāaṇtisāukumāaṛyaṣwarāaṛthināaṃ
Ḳśaṭṣ̌ēeṇaparēesaṛpaśaṣtrāagniglpitāaṭmanāaṃ
Vāatapiṭtaviṣōṇmāadaśōśāalaḳśmēejẉarāapaḥaṃ *(As. Su 6/73-74)*

intake of milk and *ghēe* is the best nourishing and refreshing combination.

Ghēe that is 10 years old is called '*purāan*'; 100 years old *ghēe* is called *Kuṃbhghrit* and *ghēe* that have been aged for more than a century is called '*mahāghrit*'.

Despite having strong odour, mature *ghēe* cures mental illness, intoxication, fainting, malaria, and cataract. It also cleans and heals wounds[482].

8. Oil

Oil comes next in line to *ghēe* among the most beneficial oily substances. Earlier the word oil was used only for sesame oil, but now it is used to refer to all oils.

Oil normally is sweet and astringent. It spreads all over the body before being digested. It strengthens *pịtta* and physical strength, and nourishes skin. Oil lends strength, stability and nourishment to muscles; sharpens intelligence, boosts digestion, and binds waste products. It clears the vaginal passage. Oil is considered the most potent of all *vāyu* calming substances. On being mixed or heated with herbs, it acquires their medicinal properties. Hence, oil proves to be a very effective medicinal and curative substance[483].

Body massages using a variety of oils calms *vayu* aggravation, relives fatigue and wards off signs of old age. It clears vision, softens the skin lending it a glow, keeps away wrinkles, strengthens the body and encourages sleep. Oiling hair relieves headache and counters balding, premature graying and hair loss[484].

Oil extracted from different materials like sesame, mustard, coconut, linseed has different properties[485]. They have been described in brief here.

Oil has a peculiar tendency: while it helps a thin person gain weight, it also helps an

---

482. *Purāaṇaṃ timiraṣ́wāasapēenasajwarakāasanuṭ*
Mōoṛchhāa kuṣ́thaviṣ́ōṇmāadagrahāapaṣmāaranāaśanaṃ (Su. Sū 45/108)
Purāaṇaṃ jayati vyāadhēeṇ vṛiṇaśōdhanaṛōpaṇaṃ
Pōoṛvāaṇkṭāaṇṣ́chāadhikāaṇ kuṛyāaḍ guṇāaṇṣtadaṃritōpamaṃ

483. *Vāataghnēṣōoṭtamaṃ balyaṃ ṭwachyaṃ mēdhāagnivaṛdhanaṃ*
Tāilaṃ saṇyōgāsaṇṣkāarāaṭ saṛvarōgāapahaṃ mataṃ
Tīlaṃ ṗrayōgāadajarāa niṛvikāarāa jitaṣ́ramāaḥ
Āashnati balāaḥ saṇkhyē dāityāadhipatayaḥ parāa (AS Sū 6/77)

484. *Aḅhyaṇgō vāatahāa puṣ́ṭtiṣwapnadāarḍrthayabrihaṭwakriṭ*
Dagdnabhagnakṣ́aṭarōojāakḷamṣramajarāapahaḥ
Rathāakṣ́acharmaghaṭavaḍ bhavanṭyaḅhyangatō guṇāaḥ
Ṣpaṛśanē5ḅhyadhikō vāayuḥ ṣpaṛśanaṃ ċho ṭwagāaṣrayaṃ
Ṭwaċhyaṣ́ċh paramaḅhyaṇgō yaṣtvāaṭ taṃ śēelayēdataaḥ
śirahṣravaṇāpāadēṣu tāṃ viśeṣeṇa śēelayēṭ
Sa kē ṣ́yaḥ sēelitō mōoṛdhani kapāalēṇḍriyatarpaḥah (A.S.Sū 3/56-59)

485. *Tāilaṃ ṣwayōnivaṭtatra makḥyaṃ tēekṣ́ṇaṃ vyavāayi ċha*
Ṭwagdōśakṛidachakṣ́u ṣ́yaṃ sōokṣ́mōṣ́ṇaṃ kaphakṛiṇṇa ċha (A.S.Sū 6/99)

overweight person reduce fat. Being liquid/ fluid, it easily reaches the *srotas*. The *srotas* of a thin person are shriveled[486]. Oil enters these and opens them, making it possible for food to provide wholesome nourishment to the body. Similarly, it penetrates the *srotas* of an overweight person, and reduces the fat deposited in and around them. Modern medical science also does not consider oil bad for obesity, diabetes, heart-problems etc.

Oil shows another unique quality. It can cause as well as relieve constipation because it both, binds stool, and expels loose stool.

♦ Sesame Oil[487]

Sesame oil is the most superior of all oils. It is used both externally (for massage) and internally (as a part of diet). It is pungent, heavy, hot, cool to touch, nourishing, and spreads easily in the body. It lends strength, stability and lightness, boosts digestion, sharpens intelligence and cleans the uterus. It cures loose motions, injury, urinary disorders, head and uterus pain and ear problems, calms *vāyu-kapha* and binds waste products. When it is taken internally, it might prove harmful for skin, heart and eyes, but external use of sesame oil is beneficial for all these body parts.

Sesame oil is also used to cure wounds, sprains, burns and fractures. It is used for inhalation, fomentation, massage and as ear drops. It can also be used to cook food. Sesame oil does not increase *kapha* despite being oily. It also calms *piṭta* when used for massage.

♦ Mustard Oil

Bitter in potency and touch, mustard oil is light but hot and pungent. Besides reducing *kapha-vāyu* and semen, it also vitiates *piṭta* and blood. On the other hand, it boosts digestion and cures skin problems, head and ear disorders, and destroys worms. Mustard oil is very beneficial for people suffering from spleen enlargement[488].

---

486. Ḳriśāanāaṃ ḅrihaṇṇāayāalaṃ śthōolāanāaṃ kaṛśanāaya cha
Baḍḍhviṭakaṃ ḳrimighnaṃ cha saṇṣkāarāaṭsaṛvarōgajiṭ (A.S.Sū 6/100)

487. Tāilaṃ ṭwāagnēyamuśṇaṃ tēek ṣnaṃ madhuraṃ madhurvipāakaṃ
briṇhaṇaṃ ṗrēeṇaṃ vyavāayi sōok ṣma viśadaṃ guru saraṃ vikāasi
ṿri ṣyaṃ ṭwakṗrasāadanaṃ śodhanaṃ mēdhamāaṛdavamāaṛdavamāaṃsa ṣthāiṛya
vaṛṇabalakaraṃ chak ṣu ṣyaṃ baḍdha mōotraṃ lēkhanaṃ tiḳtakaṣāayāanu
rasaṃ pāachanamanilabalāasak ṣyakaraṃ ḳrimighnaṃasiṭapiṭtajananaṃ
yōniśirah̩ kaṛṇaśōola ṗraśamaṇaṃ gaṛbhasyāśōdhanaṇcha̩
Tathāa c̣hhiṇṇabhiṇṇaviḍdhōṭpi ṣṭac̣hyuṭamathitak ṣatapiṇchitabhagna
Ṣrutitaḳśāarāa g̣nida g̣dha vi ṣli ṣṭadāaritāaritāabhihataduṛbhagnaṃriga
ṿyāalavida ṣṭaṗraḅhritiṣu cha pariṣēkāaḅhyaṇgavagāahāadiṣutila tāilaṃ
ṗraśaṣyate (Su. Sū 45/112)
Taḍvaṣtiṣuc̣ha pāanēṣu naṣyē kaṛnāaḳśipōoraṇē
Aṇhapāanavidhāu chapi ṗrayōjyaaṃ vāataśāaṇtayē (Su. Sū 45/113)

488. Kaṭōo ṣṇaṃ sāaṛṣapaṃ tāilaṃ raḳtapiṭta ṗradōoṣaṇaṃ
Kaphaśukrāanilaharaṃ kaṇdōokōthavināaśanaṃ (Ch. Sū 27/290)
Kaṭōo ṣṇaṃ sāaṛṣapaṃ tēek ṣaṇaṃ kaphaśuṛāanilāapahaṃ
laghupiṭṭāaṣraḳriṭkāatha ku ṣthāa śāuvraṇajaṇtuji (A S. Sū 6)

♦ Groundnut Oil

This oil is hot, heavy, and oily, destroys *kapha-vāyu*, and increases *piṭta*. Massaging it on skin causes dryness. It is a very popular cooking medium these days.

♦ Coconut Oil

This oil is used instead of *ghēe* in southern parts of the country. It is heavy, cool, *vāyu-piṭta* destroying, increases *kapha* and nourishes hair. It is the best oil for hair.

♦ Linseed Oil[489]

This oil is sweet-sour, hot, has bitter after taste, vitiates *piṭta* and blood, destroys *vāyu* and causes skin problems.

9. Honey

There are different types of honey. Though it is typically brown, it can range from yellowish to red to black. Usually it is astringent-sweet, cool, rough, and heavy, and calms *kapha*, toxins, bleeding, thirst and hicups . It relieves congestion, heals wounds, and is beneficial for people suffering from urinary disorders, leprosy, nausea, breathlessness, diarrhoea, worm, cough. Honey increases *vāyu*, heals and cleans wounds. Some experts like *Sushrut* believed that honey had a calming effect on the three *doshas*[490].

New honey is nourishing, destroys *kapha* when taken in small quantities. Old honey cures constipation and helps reduce fat. Honey acquires and enhances qualities of other herbs that it is used with. Therefore honey is used a lot with *ayuṛvedic* medicines.

Honey and heat are considered opposing forces. Hence it should not be taken with hot substances, during summers and ailments caused due to heat. The only condition heated honey should be used is during administering purgation through vomiting. As the heated honey is eliminated from the body, it does not cause any harm[491].

Taking honey and *ghēe* in equal quantities should be avoided.

---

489. *Āaturaṣyaṃ madhurāamlaṃ tu vipāakē kaṭukaṃ tathāa*
U ṣṇavēeṛya hitaṃvāatē raktapittapṛakōpanaṃ (Ch. Sū 27/292)
Umāakusuṃbhajaṃ sōṣaṃ ṭwagdōśakaphapittakṛit (A. S. Sū 6/104)

490. *Vāatalaṃ guru śēetām cha raktapittakaphāapaham*
Saṇdhāaṭriçhchhēdanaṃ rōokṣyaṃ kaṣāayaṃ madhuraṃ madhu
Chakṣuṣayaṃ çhhēdi triṭślēṣmaviṣāahidhma5ṣrapittaṇut (Ch. Sū 27/245)
Kuṣthamēdhaḳrimiçhçhhardiśwāasakāasāatisāarajiṭ
Vṛaṇa śōdhanaṣaṇdhāanarōpaṇaṃ vāatalaṃ madhu
Rōokṣa kaṣāayamadhuraṃ taṭtulayāa madhuśaṛkarāa (A.S.Sū 6/91-92)

491. *Haṇyāaṇmadhōośṇamuśṇāartamathavāa ṣaviṣāaṇvayāaṭ*
Gururōokṣakaṣāayaṭwāaçhhāiṭyāaçhchāalpaṃ hitaṃ madhu (Ch. Su 27/246)
Uśṇamuśṇāartamuśṇē ça yukaṃ chōsṇāirnihanti tat
Viṣāaṇvayaṭwēna viṣapuśpēḅhyō5pi yatō madhu (A.S. Sū 6/93)

Chapter 7

Unfavourable Food and Useful Combinations

In the previous chapter it has been explained that the way wholesome or useful foods take care of human health and keep diseases away, in the same way non-wholesome and non-useful foods harm health and invite diseases. Non-wholesome foods are of several kinds. Some of the foods are non-wholesome by their nature and create problems on consumption; they may even cause diseases and at times create heaviness in body. Some of these by their nature are beneficial when consumed alone, but become harmful when taken along with other things or taken at particular time, season or cooked with certain other food items. In this way they may become the cause of several diseases. Such foods cause imbalance in the constituents of useful body secretions, blood cells and tissues. They do not allow wastes generated in digestion, metabolism etc. to be eliminated smoothly. In this way problems, at times serious ones, develops in the body and diagnosis of the cause becomes difficult. Prolonged use of such unfavorable food affects the health of an individual by disturbing normal body tissues. This condition may cause diseases like leprosy, leucoderma, blindness, anaemia, acidity, fever, thyroid, debility, sexual disorders, epilepsy, oedema, deformity in offspring, fistula, pinus, *visarp,* colitis *(grahani),* indigestion *(mandagani),* dry ginger *(shoth),* boil or cruption *(visfot)* etc. At times it may cause death also. Unfavorable foods are of several kinds viz:

1. Unsuitable diet for an area – consuming water dominated foods in humid areas and cold foods in cold areas
2. Unsuitable diet for a season – eg. cold, rough and light food in winter
3. Unsuitable diet for a digestive power – eg. heavy, oily and sweet food being consumed by a person with weak digestive powers
4. Quantity – eg. taking *ghēe* and honey in equal quantities
5. Unsuitable diet for a habit – eg. wheat being consumed by a person used to eating rice everyday
6. Unsuitable diet for a *doshas* – eg. person with *vāyu* dominated constitution eating *vāyu* aggravating diet
7. Unsuitable diet for a *sanskaar* and digestion *(pāak)*(tradition) – eg. eating sour foods from copper vessel
8. Unsuitable diet for a potency – eg. eating hot and cold potency foods together. For eg. orange, pineapple etc. with milk, curd, buttermilk etc.
9. Unsuitable diet for a waste elimination - eg. people suffering from constipation, those passing hard and dry stool, suffering from gas formation consuming light and *vāyu* aggravating foods. Similarly people with easy stool elimination consuming heavy foods in large quantities.
10. Unsuitable diet for a body condition – eg. heavy and oily foods by obese

people, dry and light foods by the anorexic.

11. Unsuitable diet for a time – eg. Eating before morning ablutions, eating when not hungry, not eating when hungry, etc.
12. Unsuitable diet as per healthy diet principles – eg. breaking rules regarding food habits. Drinking cold water after *ghēe* (*ghēe* must always be followed by hot/warm drinks), exercising after a meal, not drinking cold water after food containing wheat etc.
13. Unsuitable diet for a cooking – eg. uncooked food, food cooked in bad medium or on impure/polluted source of heat.
14. Unsuitable diet for a combination – eg. combining wrong foods like sour things with milk.
15. Unsuitable diet for a taste – eg. forcefully eating food that is disliked
16. Unsuitable diet for qualities/properties – eg. food without taste essence or bad taste essence
17. Unsuitable as per classic texts - eg. Foods taken as against *Achar samhita*'.

Some harmful combinations are listed below:

Milk with	curd, salt, radish, radish leaves, salad, garlic, sahijan, ajark, tamarind, musk melon, papaya, Bengal quince *(belfal)*, cocunut, *āmrātak*, *ambāda*, lemon, *neekuch*, *karōuṇda*, banana, *kamrakh*, black berry, *kaith*, *paṛawat*, pomegranate, gooseberry, *galgal*, *Lufta acutangula* a gourd *(torai)*, jaggery, sesame cake, *Kulthi*- a type of pulse, black gram, moth, *niśhpāav*, *kaṇgu*, *vanak*, flour of wheat gram *(sattu)*, oil, sour foods, fish.
Curd with	milk pudding, milk, cottage cheese, hot foods, hot meals, musk melon, *tāad* fruit
Milk Pudding with	gruel, jackfruit, sour foods, flour of wheat gram *(saṭtu)*, alcohol etc.
Honey with	Black night shade *(makoi)*, *ghēe*, rain water, lotus seed, radish, warm water, warm milk and other warm foods, Saffron flower *(kusumbh)* leaves, asafoetida leaves, atrocarpus laucha fruit, syrup *(āasav)* made of *shaarkar* and dates.
Cold Water with	*ghēe*, oil, warm milk and warm things, watermelon, guava, cucumber, groundnut, *chilgozāa* (pine tree fruit).
Warm Water and other Drinks with	Honey, marking nut *(bhilāwā)*.
Ghee with	equal amount of *ghēe*, cold water, atrocarpus laucha fruit *(Neekuch)*.
Musk Melon with	Garlic, curd, milk, radish leaves.

Water Melon with	Cold water, mint.
Rice with	Vinegar
Atro-carpus *Laucha* Fruit with	Black gram, jaggery, *ghēe*, honey, milk, curd
Kameela with	Butter milk
Sesame Paste with	Poi Shak *(Upodikā)*
Kśhār with	Prolonged use
Salt with	Excessive and prolonged use
Mustard Oil with	Turmeric *(Haariḍrik)* leaves
Sprouted Pulses with	Lotus stem
Black Night shade *(Makoi)* with	Long and black pepper, jaggery, honey, fish
Black Gram with	Radish
Banana with	Buttermilk
Long pepper *(Pippali)* with	Fried Fish
Ghee with	Kept in brass container for more than 10 days
Milk with	Wine *(Sura)*, gruel *(khichdi)*

Eating the wrong combinations leads to imbalance in the body resulting in various disorders.

Non Vegetarian combinations that need to be avoided are:

Fish	milk
Pigeon meat cooked in mustard oil	honey, milk
tame *(Gramya)*/wild *(anoop)*/ water animals *(jalchar)*	honey/*sesame*/milk/raddish/
Birds and animals	blackgram/lotus stem/sprouts
Parakeet bird	mustard oil/honey/ cooking, roasting, grinding on wood of turmeric
Crane meat	Three Leaved ceper *(vāarooni madya)*, *kulmāaśh*, roasting in pig fat
Peacock meat	cooking in airand oil, on Ricinus communis Linn. (Castor oil plant) *(Airand)* wood
Cooked in fish oil	long pepper
Bhāas meat	roasted on coal
Pork	hot foods

Some examples of beneficial combinations

Certain food items, when eaten in combination, enhance each others' qualities and provide excellent nutrition. Effects of overeating can be negated if it is followed up by a food item that counters the effect. A brief list of such combinations is given below:

Food Item	Food Item That Helps Digestion
Black gram	buttermilk,
Bengal gram	Radish
Green gram	Gooseberry (Amla)
Arhār	Fermented water (kanji)
Kulthi	Oil
Wheat	Cucumber
Corn	Thyme
Kodo	*Piṇdālōo*
Shyamak/*talwarp phal)* type of bomboo *(nēevar)*, *kāaṇgi, kodo, moth*	Curd water
Gruel *(khichdi)*	Rock salt
Piṭthi *(paste)*	Cool water
Black gram *pitthi* preparations	Neem root
Milk	Greengram soup
Ghēe limonum *(Jaṃbīrī)*	Citrus medica var Lemon juice
Buttermilk made from cow milk	Lukewarm rice water
Buttermilk made from buffalo milk	Rock salt
Curd made from buffalo milk	Shell ash
Coconut	*bhāat* (rice)
Mango	milk

Food Item	Food Item That Helps Digestion
Banana	*Ghēe*
Orange	*Jaggery*
Atrocarpus lauch (Badhal)	Banana
Citrus medica var limonum *(Jaṃbīrī)* lemon	Salt
Grape fruit, Pista, walnut, almond	Clove
The lemon of india snaveolens (parhal-Hindi) bitter gourd, pumpkin, bamboo sprout *(aṇkur)*	*Kśhar* water of *Palāaśh*
Potato	Rice water
Yam	Jaggery
Pindaloo	*kodo*
Scripus grossas (Kseroo)	Dry ginger
Kśhar	buttermilk
Salt	Rice broth *(dhowan)*
Miśhri	Dry ginger
Jaggery	Dry ginger and sweet grass cyprus
Sugar cane	Ginger
Curd mixed with sugar and spice	*Trikuti*

Important Diseases and Their Treatment

Every disease has been explained in detail in *Ayuṛved*. For their treatment several medicines have been suggested. These medicines are combinations of different herbs and other substances. For important ailments particular herbal combinations have been suggested in detail. Important drug/medicine combinations suggested in *Ayuṛved* are listed below for the benefit of readers.

Disease	Important herbs/medicines
All kinds of fever	Nut grass *(Nāgar motha),* *Indica fumitory (Piṭtapda)*
Excessive Thirst	Heat soil cloth in fire, cool it in water, and drink this water
Vomiting	*Khēel/lājā*
Urinary disease	*Shilajeet*
Diabetes	Gooseberry *(Āmlā),* Turmeric
Anaemia	Wheat, fresh juice
Vāyu, Kaph	Myrobalan *(Harad)*
Liver & Spleen Ailments	Long pepper *(Pippali)*
Bone fracture	*Lakh lauifer tuchardia (Lac)*
Poison	*Albizzia Lebbek (Shirish)*
Obesity and excess *vāyu*	Hook ex stocks *(Guggul)*
Wound-healing, TB., Leprosy	Guggul, *Trifla,* Myrobalan *(harad),* Belliric myrobalan *(bahedā),* Gooseberry (Āmlā)
Skin diseases	Malabar nut *(Adūsa)*
Diarrhoea	*Holarrhena antidysenterica (Kutaj) (kudha)*
Piles, deadly skin ailments	*Vakayan*
Vish rog (Poison), Heart Ailment	Purified pearl dust *(Moti Aṛjun)*
Obesity	*Trifla*, Rasāaṇjan Winter cherry *(Aṣhwagaṇdha)*

Disease	Important herbs/medicines
Worms (stomach)	*Embelia ribes Burm. f. (Vayvidang)*
Weakness due to T.B.	Goat milk, Butter
Gout	Giloy, Nut grass *(Nāgar Motha)*
Grahni	Butter milk
Leprosy (kushath)	khadir /*khair* Juice
Madness/pagalpan	old *ghēe* of cow
Epilepsy (Mirgi)	Indian Pennywort *(bṛāḥmi)*
Insomnia	Buffalo milk, Indian spikenaral *(Jatāmānsi)*
Pulse related ailment, gastric/*vāyu*	Garlic
Paralysis	Crude sugar (*deśhi khānd*) + butter
Stomach ailment (Oedema & others)	Camel milk, ginger, leadwort *(chiṭrak)*
Indigestion, problem in passing urine	*Pāśāṇbhed, Gokhru*
Bronchitis, cough Headache and other	*Kaṇṭkāri/kateli*
Skull problem	Nasal medicine *(Naṣya)*
Mouth/buccal ailment	Nasal medicine *(Naṣya)* and oral medication *(kaval gṛah)*
Numbness	Fomentation
Boil	Blood- letting
Eye ailment	*Naṣya* and *Aṇjan*
Stiff body/ *parshvshool*	Pond *(Pokhar)*
Fatigue	Bathing
Gastric/*vāyu*	Enema, oil
Acidity	Virechan/*daṣt*, *ghēe*
Kaph	Vomit, honey
Ayu ki sthirtha	Gooseberry *(Amla)*

Disease	Important herbs/medicines
Induction of body resistance	Exercise (*yoga &pranayam*)
Joint Pain (*Vataj rog*)	*Rāasna*
Indigestion	Myrobalan *(Harad)*
Piles, Shooting pains	Root of Leadwort *(chitrak)*
Chest pain , asthma, cough, hiccup	*Pokhar*
Bleeding from mouth, nose etc	Pineapple

Effects of Some Foods and Medicines on Human Health

Foods and Medicines	Effects On Health
Balanced diet	Maintains prolonged good health
Frequent water intake	Balanced body
Milk	Energetic body
Salt	One of the best food taste providers
Sour substance	Provides good taste
Honey	Calms Kaph- piṭta dosha
Ghēe	Calms vata- piṭta dosha
Sesame oil	Calms vata- Kaph dosha
Vomit (Vaman) treatment	Best Kapha reliever
Purgatory (Virechan) Treatment	Best piṭta reliever
Enema (Basti) Treatment	Best vāyu reliever
Fomentation (Swedan) Treatment	Best body softener
Physical exercise	Best way to make body strong/solid
Goat Milk	Best during anorexia, calms bleeding and increases breast milk

Foods and Medicines	Effects On Health
Buffalo milk	Best to induce sleep
Cane Juice	Increases urine quantity
Barley	Increases stool quantity
Jamun	Inceases *vāyu*
Sheep Milk	Increases *Kapha* and *piṭta*
Black gram	Increases *Kapha* and *piṭta*
Gavedhuk Food	Reduces weight
Kulthi	Takes care of acidity
Madan fal	Vomit inducing
Trivrat (*niśhoḍh*)	Best in Purgation
Guava	Best in light purgation *(Virechan)*
Pigeon pea *(Snuhi/thuhar)*	Best in severe purgation *(Virechan)*
Apāmārg	Best in Removal of *Kaph* etc from head
Gooseberry *(Amla)*	Revitaliser *(Rāsāayan)*
Root of Castor	Aphrodisiac and reaction *(parku-piṭta)* correction
Mustha/ *Nāgar motha*	Improves digestion, checks loose motion, Helps in movement of air in intestine downwards
Shayonak Udīchay	Soothing body, appetite improvement, stops Vomiting, loose motion, gastroentitis
Bengal quince *(Bilv/bel)*	Calms *vata Kaph*, improves digestion, strength
Tivisha/*atēes*	Relief in *vāyu*, *Kapha*, *piṭta,* improves digestion, Stops gastroentitis, provides strength
Lotus, Utpal/Kumud	Bleeding, weakness
Duṛalbhā	*Piṭta* & *kaph* treatment
Kutaj/Kudha	Treatment of aggravated *kaph*, *piṭta*, profuse bleeding, weakness

Foods and Medicines	Effects On Health
Priyangu *Kaśhmaṛya/gaṃbhari*	Stops profuse bleeding
prashinparni	Improves digestion, aphrodisiac, blood treatment of *vāyu dosha*
Bala	Gas/*vāyu* problem, provides strength and virility
Shalparni	Calms down *tri-dosha,* sexual stamina *(Vajikaran)*
Asfoetida (*Hēeng)*	Takes care of *vayu* & *kapha dosha*, helps in downward movement of air in stomach, helps in digestion and removal of extra fat deposits
Amalvet	Calms down *vayu* and *kaph*, digestive
Barley ash	Piles treatment, removal of vomit sensation and gastric condition
Regular butter milk	Useful in treatment of wrongly treated consumption patients of colitis *(Grāhni)*, swelling *(sujan)*, piles *(bawāsir)*/piles, *sneh*
Consumption of Milk and *Ghēe*	Best rejuvenator
Ghēe+ roasted barley flour in equal	Aphrodisiac, virility
Gargling with sesame oil	Strengthen teeth, taste to food
Pack Sandal paste	Removes undesirable, foul body smell
Pack *Agaru* and *Raasna*	Provides pleasing coolness to body
Lāamijak, Uśhēer	Helpful in controlling of excess sweat, and prevention of skin ailment.
Massage with *Kusht*/and *pulits*	Checks *Vāyu* faults *(Vikar)*/ailment
Liquorice root (*Mulāihti)*	To improve eye sight, voice, hair shine; aphrodisiac, improvement in healed skin color

Foods and Medicines	Effects On Health
Fresh Air Environment	Refreshes by removing fatigue
Diet as per digestive power	Improves digestion.
Overeating	Causes severe indigestion
Eating on time	Maintains health
Eating before digestion of previous meal	Causes duodenum ailments
Irregular eating	Results in abnormal digestion
Delaying urination and excretion	Extremely harmful
Mental peace	Eessential to remain disease free
Happiness	Pleasant emotional state
Unhappiness	Destroys vitality
Working beyond capacity	Reduces life span
Celibacy	Increases longevity
Promiscuity	Effects longevity
Intercourse during menses	Worst, condemned deed
Depression	Invites diseases

Chapter 9

Stages of Life and Rejuvenation-Therapy

The average age of a human being, according to our *shastras/* ancient texts, is nearly one hundred years. The following ten attributes have been considered essential for a happy and healthy life:

1. *Bālya* (innocence)	tenderness
2. Growth	growth of body
3. Splendour/brilliance	energy and vitality
4. Wisdom	power of judgement
5. Lustre/glow	Healthy soft skin
6. Vision	power of seeing
7. Sperm/ovum	life power
8. Power/valour	courage
9. Intelligence	power of knowledge
10. Motor organs (mobility)	power to move motor organs

According to our ancient saints, in the absence of the above attributes, there is no happiness. Deficiency or absence of these elements makes the human body vulnerable to a host of diseases.

The human life span is divided into four stages:

1. Infancy childhood: till 16 years .
2. Youth and middle age: 17 to 60 years

This stage has been divided in three sub- stages

A. Development Period	B. Youth	C. Self sufficient period
17 to 20 years is the period of fast development of *dhatus* in body organs.	21 to 40 years. Characterised by energy, vitality and full potency of all *dhatus* and sense and motor organs.	41 to 60 years. Not much growth but stability in energy and strength of previous period.

D. **Old age:** 61 to 100 years.Gradual degeneration of all tissue elements sets in, leading towards death.

As explained above, between 41 to 60 years is the stage of stability. But it is possible only when during this period one takes nutritious and balanced diet, manages physical, mental and other stress, anxiety etc. to maintain the quality of health similar to pre-forty years period. One should follow daily and seasonal routines as recommended in *Ayurved* taking into consideration the wholesomeness and deficiencies of the eatables and other requirements of the body.

Otherwise one is not likely to maintain even normal health. Because there is no growth of tissues/cells during this period, the tissue growth of the previous period is to be maintained according to daily and seasonal to rules of *Ayurved* and not allowed to deteriorate at any cost. The slightest carelessness in matters mentioned above would take a servious toll on health. Generally, in this period of life one is occupied with different thoughts and deeds in diverse fields. The wisdom to take appropriate decisions is at its peak during this period. Deviation from the ideal path, working against the conscience, lust, greed for wealth, fame etc. destroys peace and one loses physical, mental, spiritual power to work. Some people indulge in excessive sex. This makes them weak. Such people develop wrinkles on their face, grey hair, baldness and other signs of old age. Comparatively, there is reduction in their appetite, digestion power and productivity.

Diet during this age should be decided keeping the above in mind. At this age, exposure to severe winter, summer, rain etc. should be avoided as vulnerability to seasonal illnesses increases. During this period there is deposition of fat on different parts of body particularly stomach, neck, face, thighs, buttocks, limbs etc. and one may look fat or obese. This indicates defective metabolism in the body.

It is clear that the energy generated in the body due to diet and other sources declines during this period. This clearly indicates that regulating diet and life-style is crucial to maintaining good health and keeping in shape till 60 years of age.

After attaining an age of 60 years, the ageing phase of human body begins. Despite all efforts, the body begins to show signs of ageing. Digestive power gets eroded. Waste products start accumulating in the body. Nutritive and balanced food also does not help in preventing weakness in the body. Eyesight starts deteriorating. Calcium accumulation in the body is on the increase. Synovial fluid in the joints starts drying causing rigidity and loss of elasticity. This is the cause of pains in joints, arthritis, cervical spondilitis etc. The nervous system becomes somewhat rigid and does not work properly. Memory loss occurs. Hearing is also impaired. Nerves and arteries loose their elasticity and tenderness. Heart, kidneys, lungs and other vital organs of the body lose their original strength and efficiency. These changes lead to high blood pressure, insomnia, enlargement of prostrate glands etc. Pancreas becomes incapable of secreting enough insulin leading to diabetes. Fractures during this age take longer to heal as setting of bones becomes difficult. Eyesight is affected by cataract. Gums become weak and teeth start to decay and fall. In brief, an individual at this age becomes helpless physically and mentally. He/she becomes a sort of liability for himself, his family and the nation. His/her life becomes boring and unhappy.

In old age, the rejuvenation therapy documented in *Ayurved*, is of great help. The objective of this therapy is to maintain proper digestion and keep it normal as far as possible. Normal digestion promotes multiplication of cells/tissues. These tissues provide energy to the body. Rejuvenation therapy provides strength to nerves and nervous system. This provides unctuousness, tenderness and elasticity to joints and body organs. It maintains proper mind and body balance. Rejuvenation therapy helps in protection against the disease and disorders of old age. By under-going rejuvenation therapy during old age, one can hear and see properly. The shine on the face is restored. Skin remains smooth and maintains lustre of youth. Nerves, veins and arteries remain fairly healthy and strong. Brain and body tissues remain active. One can remain young for a longer period if not throughout life. Physical and mental faculties remain strong and co-ordinate properly. This therapy is a must for every person as it helps in building up a healthy and physically strong society.

Appropriate Time for Rejuvenation Therapy

The main aim of rejuvenation therapy is to keep diseases and disabilities of old age at bay. One should adopt /practice rejuvenation therapy as a preventive measure to old age problems prior to reaching old age, i.e. during youth or adult period itself. The medicines, exercises etc. would be fully useful because of normal functioning of digestive system and metabolic activities in the body during the youth and adult periods.

The two following conditions are to be religiously followed prior to undergoing rejuvenation therapy:

1. Cleaning of body (digestive system).

   Without clearing alimentary canal by induced vomiting and purgation one does not get full advantage of rejuvenation therapy. Hence, removing wastes from body before practicing this therapy is necersary .

2. Positive thinking and conduct.

   A person practicing this therapy should think and speak of building of good society. Such conduct and deeds help in keeping the body young even without the use of medicines. Such individuals remain lively and young. Individuals practising rejuvenation therapy should adopt a simple, vegetarian, disciplined and positive way of life. Their association and day to day dealing should be with civilized and ethical people.

Persons Suitable For Rejuvenation Therapy

An individual can be considered suitable for rejuvenation therapy if he/she has good character possessing the following qualities:

- Speaks truth and does not get angry quickly.
- Does not trouble others.
- Does not get stressed and does not resort to more than required hard work.
- Does not take alcohol and avoids sex.
- Remains composed in all situations and conditions.
- Speaks very plain and is straightforward.
- Remains hygienic and chants holy mantras.
- Possesses wisdom.
- Donates, believes in giving alms and is religious.
- Respects God, learned people, teachers, the aged and cows.
- Practises non-violence, and is kind and ethical.
- Consumes *ghēe* and milk.
- Shuns false pride, is humble, has self-control, has abiding faith in God and elders, is religious and spiritual.
- Reads religious and other holy books.
- Maintains strong character, free from social and other vices.
- One who consumes nutritive and useful foods has knowledge of medicines and foods according to season, place and country.

A person with above and other similar characteristics is stable and at peace. He/she would benefit more with rejuvenation therapy.

Methods

According to *Ayurved*, rejuvenation therapy can be used in following two ways:

Indoor/Confinement To Cottage

In this method, one who is undergoing rejuvenation therapy has to make arrangements to stay in a special type of cottage having required facilities. Those undergoing treatment cannot attend to daily professional duties. It is identical to being an indoor patient.

Outdoor/Non-Confinement

In this method one can undergo rejuvenation therapy while attending his/her routine professional duties. He/she has to take wholesome food along with medication. it is similiar to being an OPD patients. For normal people the second method is appropriate.

♦ Unwholesome Food and Diet

A person undertaking rejuvenation therapy should avoid the following:

Salty, acidic and pungent foods, oils, spoiled and left-over foods, sour *kānji* (a drink made of by preserving carrots in brine), *kodo,* type of Bomboo (nivar), grain, cottage cheese, curd, oily foods, masturbation, late hours working in night, anxiety, fear, worry and anger.

♦ Rejuvenation Medicines

There is mention of several rejuvenation medicines in *Ayurved.* The important ones are *Āmlā* (Phyllanthus emblica), myrobalan *(harad),* Tinospora Cordifolia *(giloy), brāhmi* (Bacopa monnieri), liquorice root (mulethi), Convolvulus pluricanlis *(shankhpusp),* Spreading Hogweed *(punarnava),* Indian Pennywort *(mandukparni)* are important. Some of the poisonous medicinal substances such as marking nut *(bhilāvā),* Aconite *(vatsnabh)* etc. are used in rejuvenation therapy and are purified (removal of poison) before use through special processes. Besides, mercury, sulphur, *shilajeet* and gold, minerals and metals are also generally used as rejuvenators. Before use these minerals and metals are processed in such a manner that they become compatible with blood and other body fluids. Except *shilajeet,* rest of the substances having poisonous properties are to be used scientifically in combination and not individually. Ayurvedic medicine powder *(Rasa-Bhasmo)* is also used like this.

Ayurved explains each rejuvenating substance, its processing, quantity, method and time of use, wholesomeness and abstention. Hence rejuvenation therapy should be undertaken under the supervision of an able doctor and as per scientific procedures mentioned in *Ayurved.*

Besides individual medicinal substances, there are certain preparations made by combining several herbs, metals, and minerals etc. that have medicinal and rejuvenating properties.

Examples of such combination are Ayurvedic medicine *(Brahma Rasayan), Chayvanpras, Āmlakī Rasāyan, Trifala Rasāyan* etc. Out of these *Chayvanpras* is very popular. It would be appropriate to mention it in brief how it should be used in rejuvenating therapy.

♦ *Chayvanpras*

Chayvanpras is considered more of a tonic than medicine.

Method of Use and Quantity

As ejuvenating medicine, two big teaspoonfuls (total 30 gram) of *Chayvanpras* should be taken with cow milk on an empty stomach twice a day. The therapy should be started with one small teaspoonful and its quantity should be increased gradually. It should be taken for a longer period to take full advantage. The quantity and period of its use depends on the age, physical and mental condition of the patient. This herbal preparation does not have any side effects but if it is consumed in large quantity all of a sudden, it can weaken digestion resulting in loss of appetite.

♦ Wholesome and Unwholesome Diet

If milk, milk products and *ghēe* made of cow milk are taken with *Chayvanpras*, its medicinal effect increases. Sour foods like curd etc. should not be taken with *Chayvanpras*.

To avoid obesity as a result of improvement in digestion, use of foods rich in fats and carbohydrates should be minimised. Use of *Sandhav* salt in place of common salt increases medicinal effects of *Chayvanpras*. While using this and other rejuvenating medicines one should observe *Brahṃcharya*. This would speed up and enhance fruitfulness of the process.

As stated earlier, sour and bitter substances should be avoided when *Chayvanpras* is being used for rejuvenation therapy. Salt should be taken in very small quantities. As far as possible, the patient should avoid anxiety and worry. Avoiding sex would be useful.

♦ *Harad* (Myrobalan) As Rejuvenator

Badī harad (myrobalan) is also a good rejuvenating substance. Its fruit after removal of seed is used as medicine. This fruit is powdered and used as follows for rejuvenation.

Season	Taken with
Rainy	Rock salt
Winter	Sugar
Hemanṭ	Dry ginger powder
Shishir	Powder of long pepper
Spring	Honey
Summer	Jaggery/Raw sugar

One teaspoon (5gms) powder of *harad* with equal quantity of above mentioned as per season should be taken. According to the condition of the abdominal organs (stomach, intestine and bowels), the dose can be decreased or increased. Rejuvenation therapy of this kind is a unique gift of *Ayuṛved* to mankind.

No other medical science prescribes a rejuvenation therapy which is free from side effects . By practicing this therapy, a person remains healthy and happy; he enjoys a problem free old age and contributes in building a healthy and beautiful society.

Physical Strength

Good health and strong body are inseparable terms. A healthy body, in other words, is a strong body. One needs strength and energy to perform even the smallest task. In their absence, it is difficult to perform general day-to-day work. Without the required energy, one cannot face the difficult and complicated problems in life. Hence energy (strength) is an important part of a body/living being.

It is not possible to know the energy/strength of a person by merely having a look at his/her body. It is not necessary that every obese and frail person is physically strong (energetic) and weak (non-energetic), respectively. Then how is the physical strength of a person to be measured? And what is this strength/energy? It is explained here in brief.

♦ What is Energy/Strength

The final product of *ras*, blood and other *dhātus* in the body is called energy/*balshakti* strength. This energy/*shakti* is also known as oj *or ojas.* This strength nourishes all muscles and makes them stable and strong. The quality of voice and the glow of skin are determined by *ojas.* All external and internal parts of the body are able to perform their tasks well because of this strength/energy which is produced within the body.

♦ *OJ* or *OJAS*

This is a very important and vital element of the body and is dominated by the qualities of the element water. Hence it is *Saumaya* in nature. *ojas* is an elastic, oily, cold white liquid and is located in the heart. Life is dependent on it. Man lives because of it. Its absence leads to death.

ojas is the extract of the seven components of body (*dhātus*) such as blood, *ras* etc. According to *Charak Samhita, ojas* is synthesized in the body by the action of enzymes on the *dhātus* in the same way that honeybees synthesize honey from nectar collected from numerous flowers. *ojas* is white and has a yellowish tinge. It is heavy, soothing, dense, bright, sticky, and sweet. It contains all six *rasas*. Like the universe, *ojas* also contains attributes of both heat (*Agni*) and cold (*Som* or *Jal*). The *Som* component is white and the *Agni* component is yellowish red. The *Agn*i component is considered superior. When there is fall in the *Agni* component, a person becomes weak, while fall in level of *Som* leads to retention of water in the body and subsequent death.

Since there is a similarity between *kapha* and *ojas*, normal levels of *kapha* in the body build and strengthen *ojas*. On the other hand, when there is a drop in the normal levels of *kapha*, *ojas* turns into *mal* (waste toxic body products) and gives rise to several disorders.

"*Ojas* is a protective substance that vides immunity to the body. Hence *ojas* should always be maintained and nourished. It strengthens immune system. Without it, external medication is of no use. On losing *Ojas*, one becomes immune to all treatment."

Rakṣhaid balaṃ chapī niraṣya niṭyam
tadrakshitam vyadhi balṃ nihaṇti.

(Su. Ch. 18/3)

The disease commonly known as AIDS results from a drastic reduction of *Ojas* levels in the body.

The energy produced by *tej* and *ojas* is divided into three parts—*Uṭtam* (superior), *Maḍhyam* (average) and *Adham* (below average). It is also categorized as follows:

1. **Natural Energy** –This is the naturally occurring energy in the body. This is produced by *ras* and is the most superior kind.
2. **Periodic Energy**—this is the age specific energy gained during different stages of growth of human body.
3. **Acquired Energy** –This is the energy acquired through external nourishment.

♦ Characteristics Of An Energetic/Strong Person

An individual who is free from disease and ailments, displays minimum signs of ageing, completes all his tasks efficiently,takes pleasure in work, has both material and spiritual knowledge, has a strong body, is energetic and healthy.

What is a strong body? That which has more fat, muscles etc. or that which is healthy? Isn't a thin body that is relatively healthy not strong? There are several such questions. According to *Ayurved*, a person whose bones are in good shape and in the right place and distributed evenly, whose joints are strong and supple, whose organs are covered with the right amount of flesh and muscle, who is physically strong and does work efficiently, is considered to have a strong and healthy body. This is the best kind of body to have. A heavy body, which is not as capable as the previous one, is the medium type, while a body that is not well formed and lacks balance between the various components, is an inferior body. A person, whose body might look strong and healthy, but who lacks mental strength (faints on seeing blood, death, accidents and other traumatic events, or suffers from illnesses), is not considered a strong person.

♦ Problems Related To Physical Strength

A heavy body, lack of energy, numbness, sleep, fatigue, lack of efficiency, bloating, lack of muscle mass, fainting, self-pity, depression, stubbornness, blabbering- all these are related to a decrease of bodily power and energy.

The treatment for the above must be done keeping in mind the patient's strength. He must guard against fear, anger, envy, depression, self-pity, physical exercise and sexual activity. Such a patient should not indulge in activities that require a display of physical strength. Therapies, treatments, food and life-style habits that work in case of TB and chronic fever, are also recommended for these patients. Rejuvenation and semen increasing therapies must be undertaken, apart from using *vāyu* destroying oils.

Obesity and Emaciation

A person with an even distribution of muscle, mass and fat, bones of the right length and stable joints, and adequate strength is a healthy and balanced person. In contrast, people with too much or too little fat are unhealthy.

Obesity - Symptoms

Too much fat accumulation on hips, stomach and chest causing them to move while walking, is a clear sign of obesity. Another symptom is a lack of increase in body strength corresponding to the increase in body mass.

The body channels of an obese person are blocked due to fat accumulation. This causes *vāyu* aggravation especially in the stomach, which in turn aggravates digestive juices. Digestion speeds up and hunger increases. Avoiding food under such conditions leads to various disorders. *Vāyu-piṭta* imbalance leads to too much fat accumulation resulting in *vāyu* related illnesses.

The life-span of obese people is generally less than normal, and their work output is also low. They are weak, sweat profusely; experience lack of hunger and thirst, body odour increases and intercourse becomes difficult.

Causes

The most common reasons for obesity are overeating, eating heavy, sweet and cold foods in excess, lack of physical exercise, absence of sexual activity, sleeping during the day, experiencing too much joy, psychological disturbances and heredity. All these conditions cause the fat to increase more than the other body building *dhātus*. Being loose, heavy and soft, fat in large quantities becomes weak and is not able to perform its functions optimally. Reduced quantity of semen makes sexual activity difficult. Excessive sweating leads to increased body odour.

Presence of *kapha* in fat and its liquid and heavy nature reduces its capacity to bear physical activity and hard work. An obese person begins to sweat very easily.

Due to increased digestive power, hunger and thirst are also aggravated.

Underweight/Thin Individuals - Symptoms

Thin or underweight individuals have sunken stomachs, thin neck and lack of body muscles. Body veins and arteries become visible. Bone joints become conspicuous. The body looks like a skeleton.

Underweight people do not have the capacity and strength to tolerate excessive eating, hunger, thirst, pain, disease and medicine. They cannot tolerate severe summer and winter. They are unable to enjoy married life. By and large such people suffer from cough, cold, bronchitis, piles, diseases and disorders of chest and stomach.

♦ Underweight - Causes

The causes of an underweight or thin body are unbalanced, non-nutritious diet, frequent fast, eating less, anxiety, worry, stress, anger, insomnia, insufficient sleep, excessive bathing, prolonged illness, excess exercise etc.

Obesity Is More Dangerous Than Emaciation

As explained above, obese and thin body both are dangerous-undesirable and harmful. Both the conditions make the body unhealthy or diseased. Obesity is more dangerous. Obesity/ overweight and underweight disorders of the body can be corrected by more or less similar ways but corrective measures of overweight are more painful and difficult for the patient. Treatment of obesity involves destruction of accumulated fat, slowing down the digestion process and reduction of *vāyu* accumulation. This is very difficult because *Brahan Chikitsa* takes care of aggravated *vāyu* and digestion power but increases fat accumulation. On the contrary, in *Laṅghan* (leading to thin condition) treatment, there is reduction in body fat but increase in air accumulation and digestion. In other words *Brahan* treatment adds fat in obese people and *Laṅghan* treatment leads to an intolerable increase in hunger.

Treatment Principles In Brief for Over/Underweight

Obesity/overweight : Heavy and *apatarpan* foods

Thin or underweight : Light and easily digestible foods

In obese persons, these foods suppress/reduce digestive power and because of *apatarpan*, quality deposition of fat is reduced. Honey and barley possess both the qualities. easy of digest *(Laghu)* and *apatarpan* foods (viz- Callicarpa macrophylla *(priyaṇgi)* and *shalak* can be mixed with other foods to make them heavy and can be given to an obese person. For example barley, wheat cooked with oil, buttermilk etc. are beneficial for obese people. Food that is light and fattening can provide strength and strengthen digestive power in a weak person. Spiked ginger lily *(Sali)*, Coriander sativum *(Dhānya)*, *Sathi* are good example of the above. Frail people can also consume heavier foods after they have been lightened by cooking eg. asfoetida, thyme, dry ginger etc can make food easy to digest. In the same way, barley and wheat cooked in butter *(GHEE)* and milk would be beneficial for frail person.

♦ Treatment Of Obesity

Obesity can be treated with *langhan* or *apatarpan*. *Laṅghan* treatment brings lightness to the body, reduces fat and thus weight. Herbs, food and other substances used in this treatment contain principally *tejas* (*agni*), *vāyu* and *āakāsh*. In *langhan* dry, rough, small,liquid and solid herbs are used.

The following measures can be adopted for such treatment.

1. Corrective (*sanshodhan*) treatment: induced vomiting, loose motion, enema, nasal (*nasya*) treatment.
2. Observing fast: take less and light food.
3. Tolerating thirst
4. Exposure to sun and fresh air
5. Physical exercise
6. Use of herbs promoting digestion

Besides *langhan*, the following treatment can be used to treat obesity.

1. Use of fat, *kapha* and *vāyu* destroying food.
2. Enema while diet is d ry and hot.
3. Use of medicated pastes
4. Use of Tinospora Cordifolia *(Giloy)*, Nut grass *(Nāgarmotha)*, Myrobalan *(Harad)*, Terminalia Bellirica *(Bahedā)* and Gooseberry *(Āmlā)*
5. Use of Ayurvedic medicinal syrup *(takrarisht)*
6. Use of honey with cold water (one spoon) in the morning and evening.
7. Taking equal quantities of *Embelica ribes Burm.* F. *(vayabidang)*, dry ginger, Ayurvedic medicine *(yavkshar)* and iron powder (*bhasma*) with honey and gooseberry powder.
8. Use *shilajeet,* an exudate of rock.
9. Bengal guince *(Bilvadī),* Ayurvedic medicine *(panchmōol)*, use of juice of like fire *(agnimay)* with eye ointment *(rasajan),* hook ex stocks *(gugal*) or honey.
10. Eating *PraŞitikā*, *Callicarpa Macrophylla (Priyangu)*, *Sahaymak*, barley *(Yavak)*, sorghum, *kodo,* green gram, pigeon pea (Cajanus cajan) with patol and Gooseberry *(Āmlā), (Phyllanthus embilica)* followed by water mixed with honey.
11. Working hard physically, mentally, some anxiety, increased sex.
12. *Trikatu* (dry ginger, black pepper and Long pepper *(Pipali), Picrorhiza Kurrooa (Kutki)*, Myrobalan, *Bahera*, Gooseberry, *Sanjan, Vayuidang, Atis, Shalparn*i, *sauvarchal, jeeva, Ajwain, Coriander Turmeric* -All mixed. in equal quantities and take 2-5 gram powder with warm water in the morning and evening.

All the above mentioned ways are of great help in overcoming obesity. Besides, obesity other ailments like heart problem, cough, cold, skin diseases, leucorrhoea etc are also cured. Improved material comforts and the consequent reduction of physical activity is responsible for wide spread obesity in recent years. Obesity breeds dangerous ailments involving vital systems of body like blood circulation, respiratory systems etc.

Preventive and curative measures of obesity listed above help to maintain good physique and health.

♦ Treatment Of Emaciation/ Underweight

To overcome the problem of extremely underweight/thin body *brāhan* or Satiating *(sanpartan)* treatment and resources/inputs are used. This type of treatment adds weight and energy to the body because of calorie rich food. Solid, semi-solid and liquid foods rich in earth and water elements are used in this treatment. Food and drinks rich in fat and proteins, carbohydrates, vitamins are used as diet besides herbs and other elements having soothing and cooling effects. Milk, *ghēe* ,cottage cheese and other milk products, sugars find dominance in diet during treatment of underweight person. Physical treatment involves frequent bathing, good sleep for long hours, maintaining a good mood and happiness, avoiding of anxiety, enema with *snigdha* medicines etc. are part of *brahan* treatment.

the problem of being underweight.

1. Sound sleep, happiness, comfortable bed, satisfaction and control over mind.
2. Avoiding anxiety, excessive sex and physical work.
3. Staying in good places, and around pleasant relatives and friends.
4. Including curd, *ghēe*, milk, sugar, parboiled rice, black gram, wheat and jaggery in meals.
5. Enema with sweet and unctuous medicines.
6. Regular body massage with oil, bathing with warm water and application of medicated unctuous *ubṭan* (pastes)
7. Use of aromatic and incense garlands.
8. Wearing white clothes.
9. Vomiting/enema at appropriate time to get rid of problematic substances from the stomach.
10. Use of rejuvenation therapy and aphrodisiac medicines helpful in production of sperm or ovum.
11. Taking balanced diet and maintaining tension-free attitude.

The above can, as stated earlier, help in overcoming problems of being underweight. In brief, avoiding anxiety, remaining happy, having sound and adequate sleep, eating *brahan* quality food and herbs are helpful for the underweight.

Golden Rules For Maintaining Health

- Sleeping on time and rising before sunrise
- Remembering good health is not restricted to physical health; emotional and psychological well-being are crucial
- 10-15 minutes of meditation after rising has a calming effect
- A wholesome diet is key to good health. Taking medication becomes redundant without it.
- Meals should be taken in peace. Meal time should be a quiet time with oneself.
- Meals should be taken on time after the previous meal has been digested.
- Consumption of curd at night and afternoon siestas (except in summers) are harmful
- Exercising is good for the body provided if it is done more than the body's potential.
- Both obesity and thinness are harmful. Obesity more so, and therefore one must guard against it.
- Never underestimate any ailment; neglecting minor illness can be very dangerous – they can aggravate into serious disorders.

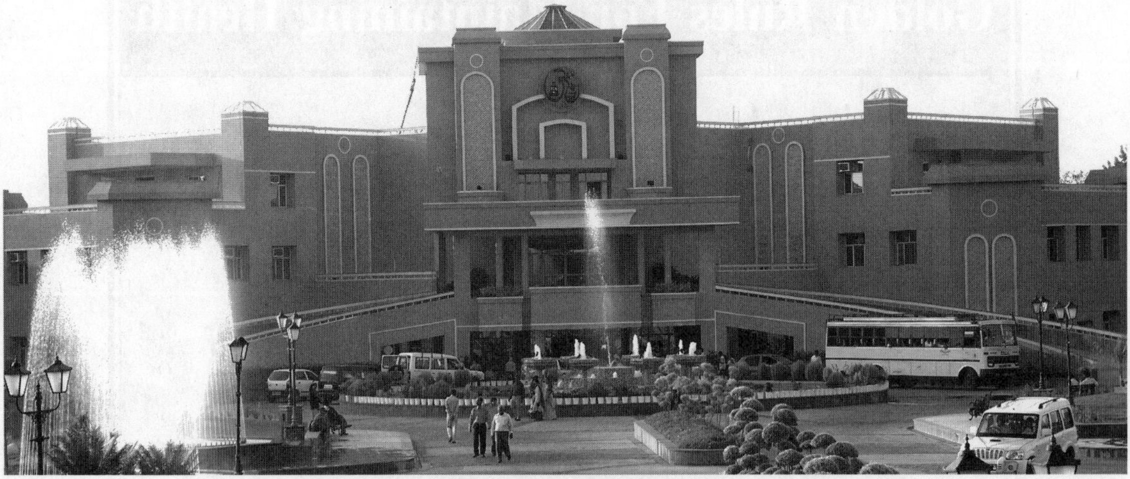

Patanjali Yogpeeth

Divya Yog Mandir Trust, Kankhal

The headquarters of *Divya Yog Mandir* Trust is located in Krupalu Bagh Ashram. Krupalu Bagh Ashram was established in 1932 by Shri Krupalu, who haled from warrior land, Mewad (Rajasthan). His original name was Yeti Kishore Chand. During the independence revolution Kishore Chandji played an active role in the freedom fight. He gave shelter to many revolutionaries in Haridwar. Local freedom fighter Veni Prasad was one of the main partners. Yati Kishore Chandji established the first public library in Haridwar and with hard labor collected around 3500 books and kept them in the library located in the Upper Road. He established dozens of schools in this area to give a momentum to the task of building the nation. Founder of Gurukul Kangadi Swami Shradhanandji had very good and close relations with him. Afterwards, Bal Gangadhar Tilak, Madan Mohan Malviya, Motilal Nehru, Mahatma Gandhi, Chittaranjan Das, Ganesh Sahankar Vidyarthi, V.J.Patel, Hakim Ajmal Khan came close to him.

Yati Kishore Chand associated himself with the Banga revolutionary party and took the responsibility of the bold task of circulating 'Yugantar" and "Lokantar" newspapers published by the party in northern India. The newspaper which was published in Bengali and English was a pain in the neck for the British. The foreign Government was afraid of this newspaper, which was used for creating revolutionaries and exposing the British. Yati Kishore Chand used to post these newspapers all over India in envelopes, sometimes from the Chandi Pahadi in Haridwar and sometimes from the library situated in Paliwala *Dharmashala*. During these days Banga revolutionary party assassinated Lord Harding in a bomb blast. Ras Behari Bose was their leader. Yati Kishore ChandJi was given the responsibility to give shelter to Ras Behari Bose. At that time the British Government had kept a reward of Rs 3 lakhs on Ras Behari Bose. Yati Kishore Chandji gave him shelter in his *ashram* situated in the midst of forest. At that time his friend Harish Babu along with three other friends came to Haridwar and told that the Britishers have come to know of the whereabouts of Ras Behari in Haridwar or Dehradun and they could raid the area any time. Yati Kishore Chand sent him to Varanasi in Dehradun Express in the disguise of Patiala tourist. Ras Behari boarded the night train to Varanasi and in the morning a huge army of policemen herded his hut. They searched every nook and corner for him but the lion was out of his cage and reached safely to Varanasi and from there he fled to Japan. The same Yati Kishore Chand became ascetic and came to be known as Krupalu Maharaj. He published a monthly magazine "*Vishwa Gyan*" to raise the flame of independence in the dependent India. Yati Kishore Chand who was leading a life of freedom fighter and revolutionary was inspired by *Yog* and spirituality and became an accomplished *yogī*. He left this world in 1968.

Disciples of Maharajji took over the responsibility of managing the pious, revolutionary, *Yog* devotion at Krupalu Bagh *Ashram*. Shri Swami Shankar Devji is one of the bonds of this tradition, whose disciple Swami Ramdevji Maharaj has enlightened the ashram with the divine flame of *Yog*, *Ayurved*, *Vedic* Culture and made it popular in India and abroad, and the entire world. *Divya Yog mandir* Trust was established in 1995 and with this medium Swami Ramdevji Maharaj has with the help of his inseparable, well-wishers namely Acharya Balkrishanji and Swami Muktanandji, and others and has given shape to several service projects. This has left deep impact on the Indian people and as a result *Veda, Yoga* and *Ayurved* are getting better known and popular.

With the divine grace of these pious souls, crores of people are getting the benefit of physical health, mental peace, self progress, spiritual development and intelligence. He is moving ahead in the fields of Religion, Yog, Spirituality, Social Service, Education and welfare of the mankind. Even then he has no ego, and believes that we are only a medium and whatever is happening, or is going to happen is the result of God's desire and grace.

Services offered by *Divya Yog Mandir* Trust

Various services have been started by the *Divya Yog Mandir* Trust within a short period of one decade and the success story created through these services is no less than a miracle for the people who are experiencing this. The multi dimensional form which the *Patanjali Yogpeeth* is taking, the people are feeling that Swami Ramdevji is definitely blessed with some divine power. In fact all this is possible because of the pious feeling of respect, devotion towards God, determination of serving the people, and welfare of the mankind, that is on the mind of Ramdev Baba and he is always inspired and active with these feelings. A summary of the various services offered by the *Divya Yog Mandir* Trust is being given below:

Organization of Yog Practice and Yog Healing Camps

Under the supervision of Revered Swami Ramdevji, the *Yog* Devotion and *Yog* Medication Camps organized all over the country have removed the myth that *Yog* is only a physical exercise. Revered Swamiji has provided a definite, meaningful and rational definition to *Yog* by making it the basis for physical health, curing diseases, mental peace, self progress, intelligence and spiritual progress. The devotees who are regularly practising *Yog* are experiencing the benefits of *Yog*. In these camps, education and training is given on *Aṣhṭāṅga yog*, *yam*, *niyama*, *āsana*, *prāṇāyāma*, *pratyāhāra*, *dhāraṇa*, *dhyāna* and *samādhi*. Arrangements are being made for the study, training and utility based activity of *Patañjali Yog-Sūtra* along with *Haṭha-Yog*, *Darśana*, *Upaniṣads*, *Veda*, *Charaka*, *Suśruta* and other texts. Arrangements are also being made to give practical training of *Yog*, *Ṣaṭkarma*, *Dhauti*, *Basti*, *Trāṭaka*, *Nauli* and *Kapāla-bhāti* and along with these six yogic activities meditation *Yog* and *Devotion Yog* will also be included.

Brahmakalpa Hospital

In *Brahmakalpa* Hospital along with *Ṣaṭkarma*, *Pancha-karma* (Massage, formentation, vomiting, evacuation of the bowels, *basti*), herbs and shrubs and essence -chemical based Ayurvedic Medicines, diet, digestion, indigestion, balanced celibacy and seasonal routine and daily routine are taught comprehensively and old and new diseases are cured. Acupressure, *Yog*, and *Āsana*, *Prāṇāyāma*, natural therapy training is being given free of cost and at very low costs for those who are unable to purchase these medicines due to insufficient funds.

Serious and incurable diseases like high blood pressure, diabetes, heart problems, asthma, obesity, acidity, allergy, ulcer, cervical spondylitis, sciatica, arthritis, cancer (first and second stage) and others are cured without operation.

In the process of giving an extensive form to *Brahmakalpa* Hospital in *Patañjali Yog pīṭha*, a residential hospital is also being created so that the patient can get admitted for treatment. Respected Swami Ramdevji Maharaj says that we should all try that no disease could torment us, the human beings.

Even if disease takes us over, we should first adopt *yog* and try to get over it. If medicine has to be taken we should give priority to Ayurvedic medicines because they are associated with our land, culture and nature and are totally harmless. For this purpose it is necessary to have the medicines manufactured at *Divya* Pharmacy with quality herbals. Therefore in order to produce cheap and qualitatively superior medicines *Divya Yog Mandir* Trust has established *Divya* Pharmacy in the *ashram* premises, where ethical medicines are manufactured according to the classical principles using experience of yog, ash, mud, gold, essence, chemical, *guggulu*, powder, globule, extractions, decoctions, *ghēe*, oil, iron etc. We are trying to see that the medicnes manufactured are of highest quality. Further we are providing these medicines at very reasonable prices. We are able to manufacture the medicines in limited quantity only. Many times the people are disappointed due to non-availability of the medicines.

Therefore, a plan is being finalized to expand the *Divya* Pharmacy as early as possible, so that your requirements are met.

Laboratory

Divya Yog Mandir Trust has its own laboratory. Its activities comprise of discovery of new medicines, testing the quality of herbs purchased for *Divya* Pharmacy, developing manufacturing scientific of method of medicines according to classical texts. Further information is obtained about the cultivation, to learn about new techniques researches are being carried on, latest literature is purchased on *Ayurved* for the library, special attention is paid to preservation and protection of medicinal plants, planning the commercial benefits and publishing the research work.

The laboratory has developed several self applied *yog* exercise and has established a mile stone in this area. Since hundreds of years, four medicinal plants of *ashtvarga* were not available and it was considered that these natural plants have lost their existence due to natural reasons. But due to the hard labor, deep interest and focussed devotion of the laboratory technicians, these four plants could be found in the snow clad mountains of Himalayas. A book published by the trust written on *Aṣṭavarga* mentions this discovery in detail.

Divya Medicinal Garden

A practical effort is being made in the ashram premises to preserve, conserve and increase the life promoting herbs, which are difficult to obtain and procure However, due to lack of space, this project did not receive the desired attention so far. Now ample space is available in *Patañjali Yoga-Pīṭha* for this purpose and plans are being developed on a large scale and preserved. The fresh essence of the plants and leaves and roots necessary for the medication will be taken care of in the *Divya* Medicinal Garden in the near future. Potted plants and seeds will be made available for sale.

Establishing *Divya Byre* (*Gośālā*)

The mission for the preservation, improvement and manufacture of medicines requires cow milk, cow urine, dung. Mission to preserve the Indian breed of cattle for the cow and protection of its breed is on going since long time in the ashram. Now in *Patañjali Yog-pīṭha*, it is being given a broader look, in which thousands of cows will be taken care of. The dung obtained from this will be used as compost manure or bio-technical manure so that the food grains, fruits, vegetables and milk can be made available which would be free of chemical fertilizers. Biogas will be manufactured from dung with which the daily needs of ashram will be fulfilled. The domestic breed of these cattle will be used to increase the cattle breed so that the cows can be protected.

Vedic Ritual

Agnihotra is a science in itself. Rituals have a special place in the Indian tradition in purifying the environment, balancing the atmosphere, making the seasons favourable, increasing the plants and their preservation, controlling the situation in case of drought and floods, curing some diseases, and to accomplish the religious rituals. Following this saintly tradition, rituals are performed in the ashram everyday. There is a proposal to construct a huge *yajña-śalā* (ritual room) in the premises of *Patañjali Yoga-Pītha*. Scientific research and study will be conducted on the useful aspects of the ritual.

Vedic Gurukula

A *Vedic Gurukula* is being managed in Kishangarh-Ghaseda, 8 km from Rewadi in Haryana to maintain the vedic tradition, culture, high ideals, modern education fields, which provides education free of cost, in which the poor and rural children are gaining culture and good education along with the children of higher society. There is a requirement of constructing a proper building to maximise the number of people who can obtain education.

Devotional *Ashram* situated at Gangotri

Divya Yog Mandir Trust has established an ashram in Gangotri for the devotees and to procure the rare herbs for the preservation and research of medicinal plants which are found in the Himalayan region, which needs to be given a wider form.

Establishment of *Patañjali Yog pīṭha*

Patañjali Yog-pīṭha is a multi- dimensional project of the original institution *Divya Yog Mandir* Trust, which will occupy an area of one lakh thousand hectares. It will play a major role in communication, training, research of *Veda, Yog* and *Ayurved*. This will provide hostel facility to around two thousand devotees. It will be a building containing 1500 rooms, and will be equipped with pharmacy, hospital, cattle ground, herbs nursery, *Yoga Sandeśa* and literature publishing and, sales research department, library, printing press, kitchen, *Yog* center, ritual room, and other facilities. The people coming to the premises will get pure and pious food, which will be free from L.P.G. chemical fertilizers, and pesticides. This premises will be developed like Rabindranath Tagore's *Shantiniketan* and will be fully self-reliant which will provide health, *Yog* practice, mental peace, and spiritual development to crores of people. This will take the shape of revered devotional field in the whole world. Swamiji has taken the vow to complete the multi- dimensional project worth Rs 100 crores with the co-operation of crores of devotees, which is being fulfilled with the blessings of the Supreme Soul.

The fund amount fixed by the trust for the purpose of membership of *Yog pīṭha* is as follows :

1. Founder member	**Rs. 5,00,000**
2. Patron member	**Rs. 2,51,000**
3. Life Member	**Rs. 1,00,000**
4. Dignified Member	**Rs. 51,000**
5. Respected Member	**Rs. 21,000**
6. General Member	**Rs. 11,000**

Publication of *Yog Sandeśa* (Hindi, English, Marathi, Bengali, Punjabi and Gujrati monthly magazine)

Keeping in mind the demand of thousands of devotees associated with the *Divya Yog Mandir* Trust, "*Yog Sandeśa*," a monthly magazine is being published (Hindi, English, Marathi, Bengali, Punjabi and Gujrati editions) since September 2003 with the cooperation of an experienced editorial team. The number of new readers is adding up every month which is a proof of its increasing popularity. A resolution has been made to spread *yog, Ayurved,* culture, tradition and spiritual thinking derived from saintly tradition to lakhs of readers in the near future. Besides poems, useful articles for the masses, activities of the trust, future plans and readers experiences will also be given place in the magazine. The extensive reach and circulation of a magazine within such a short time is the result of revered Swami Ramdevji Maharaj's profound influence.

Acupressure
Applying pressure on the special points situated on the body and curing various diseases by this is called acupressure.

Agni
It is Fire, one of the five fundamental elements. It is the biological fire that governs metabolism. It is similar in its function to Pitta and can be considered an integral part of the Pitta system in the body, functioning as a catalytic agent in digestion & metabolism. It is known as Fire, and is concerned with seeing, related to eyes by the action of movement.

Akasa
It is known as Ether, one of the five elements. It is concerned with sense of hearing related to the ear & is concerned with speech.

Asanas
Different postures formed by the practitioner as per the guidance of the teacher of the Asanas. These postures depend on the part having ailment or disorder.

Astang yog
Also known as Eight-fold Yoga. It is a divine science discovered by the learned saints and seers of ancient India, brought into a disciplined manner, preserved & produced by Saint Patanjali in the form of eight yogic-principles:- Yam, Niyam, Asana, Pranayam, Pratyahar, Dharna, Dhyan, & Samadhi. A person practising these is known to experience individual & social equality, physical health, intellectual awareness, mental peace & bliss of the soul.

Aum
It is the first cosmic soundless sound.

Ayurved
It is a holistic system of medicine that is indigenous to and widely practised in India. The Ayurved is a Sanskrit term meaning "Science of Life". Ayu means life and Veda means knowledge.

Ashwa Ayurved
Way of treating the diseased horses according to ayurvedic concept.

Agad Tantra
Treatment of diseases caused due to toxins.

Akashiya Diet
Diet having the Akasa (the fundamental element) as dominant part.

Apaya Diet
Diet having the water (element) as dominant part.

Apana Vayu
Downward breathing air.

Alochak Pitta
Sight related pitta.

Avalambak Kapha
Energizing and supportive natural kapha.

Anuvasana
Daily enema.

Aam Ras
Accumulated undigested portion of food within the body.

Ātma
The Soul or the master of the body.

Audbhid
Plants and material obtained from earth.

Avidahi
Exhaustion relieving, non-burning.

Anuloman
After gas-formation, it releases gas.

Adaana
Uttarayan is also known as adaana. Because sunlight becomes intense and evaporation process increases during this period.

Anupaan
Liquids taken after meal and medication.

Arogyambu
When only one fourth of original quantity left after boiling water, it is known as Arogyambu.

Anshodak
Water kept in sunlight.

Brahamacārya
Non-indulgence in sexual relation.

Bhedan
Helps to excrete both hard and dwaroop stool.

Bhrajak Pitta
Glazing Pitta.

Bodhak Kapha
Lends and sharpens perception.

Bhoot Vidya
Treatment of psychological as well as astrological ailments. .

Bal Tantra
Treatment of infants and children.

Bhagandar
Disease of the final part of alimentary canal.

Bandhs
These are the lockings which are done by holding a particular organ or movement inside the body for a prescribed time. These enhance the effect of the activity for which they are prescribed.

Brahma
It means creation. Brahma is the god of creation.

Brahmācari
The person who follows the path of celibacy.

Charak
Great Ayurvedic physician who wrote one of the classic texts of Ayurved.:- Charak Samhita.

Chitta
It is the mind, the faculty of reasoning & emotion. It has the nature of always being unstable; it can be controlled by practising certain exercises.

Chanchal
Swiftly mobile or unstable.

Chhāchha
Buttermilk made by churning curd with moderate amount of water.

Dharaseeta
When boiled water transferred to another utensil before cooling.

Dincharya
Ideal day behavioral routine.

Dakisinayana
Sun's southern hemispherical inclined transition.

Drava
Liquid nature.

Orida
Firm or compactness or strength.

Orista form
The impartial viewer form of existence.

Dosha
Each & every gross body has a certain proportional constitution of these three dosas i.e Vata, Pitta, and Kapha.

Dhatus
Each & everybody have seven different basic energy-parts of diet-taken known as Dhatus. These are seven in number and named as (Names on page 45).

Dharma
It is the state of steadiness of mind.

Dhyāna
It is concentration of mind over a thought of an object. It improves mental well-being of an individual.

Gaja Ayurved
Way of treating the diseased elephants, according to Ayurved.

Gaya Ayurved
Way of treating the diseased cows, according

to Ayurved.

Giltiyaan
Swelling of glands.

Ghot
Buttermilk made by churning curd without water.

Ghee
Purified butter made from cow's milk.

Hansodak
Water kept in moonlight.

Jala
It is known as water, one of five elements. It is concerned with taste, related to tongue by the action of procreation.

Jeevan
It means life. It is there as long as the person is alive.

Jangam
Obtained from living world either from plants or animals.

Kaaya Cikitsa
Treating bodily diseases through medications.

Kapha
It is one of the Tridosas translated as Phelgm. It is a combination of the elements water & earth. It is concerned with actions of stability, energy, lubrication, greed, forgiveness, possession.

Kledak Kapha
Moistening natured kapha.

Kharatva
Roughness.

Katu
Pungent and Sour Taste.

Kavalgrah
Daily gargling.

Kanji
Preserving carrots in brine, this drink is called Kanji.

Laghu
Tiny or Light or i.e. weightless.

Lekha
Enhancing digestion nature.

Mala
At the time of assimilation of food in each step energetic useful part as well as wastes are produced. These wastes are known as Malas, although the mala for one is useful for another one.

Mridu
Soft nature.

Madhur
Sweet nature.

Mand
Slow natured.

Mathit
Buttermilk made without butter.

Mahaghrit
Ghee older than a century.

Niraām vayu
Vayu without the aamras portion of food.

Nasya
Medication administered through nostrils.

Ojas
The essence or the energy part of the food.

Pragyapradh
Irregularities or disorders in the systems are the results of a person's previous actions alone at subtle or gross levels. Sometimes people ignore the righteous action due to strong desire (liking / disliking) or due to socio-psychic hindrances. All these type of deeds generate imbalances and destroy the equilibrium in the body are known as Pragyapradh.

Paarthiv diet
Diet dominated with the earthen element.

Prāna
It is a vital energy (life-energy) which activates

the body and mind. It is responsible for the higher cerebral functions, and the motor and sensory activities.

Pitta
It is bile, one of the Tridosa, a combination of agni and jal. It is concerned with the body heat, temperature, digestion perception, intelligence, anger, hate & jealousy.

Pacak Pitta
Digestive pitta.

Pravrisht
First rainy season of south India.

Puraan
10 year old ghee

Pranayam
It is breathing exercise and is a Yogic healing technique that can bring extraordinary balance in the consciousness. In practising Pranayam, one experiences pure being and learns the true meaning of peace & love. It has many healing benefits & also affects creativity. If can bring joy bliss into life.

Reiki
A spiritual way of healing with the help of cosmic-energy to cure various diseases. In this, healer (spiritual master) heals the patient by reaching and establishing the communication between himself and the subtle psychic levels of the patient.

Rasayan Tantra
Maintenance of good health and keeping the aging process under control.

Ranyak Pitta
Coloring, gratifying pitta.

Rooksa
Dry, rough natured.

Rajas form
Laborious and highly mobile natured.

Ratricarya
Ideal night behavioral routine.

Ritucarya
Ideal seasonal behavioral routine.

Rayoguna
Derived from the word Rayas. It is the active vital life force in the body which moves both the organic & inorganic universes. It is the dynamic movement.

Rechak
The process of exhalation of air out of the body is called Rechak.

Satvik
It means simple, plain without any show off in relation to life, or spicy in relation to food.

Salya Cikitsa
Treating bodily diseases by operating or removal of that particular body-part.

Salakya Cikitsa
Treating E.N.T. diseases.

Sankhya
A philosophical school.

Samana
Distributed evenly in the whole body.

Sadhak pitta
Connecting natural kapha or smooth nature.

Slesak kapha
Efficient or effective pitta.

Seetal
Cool in nature.

Saam uaye
Vayu mixed with aamras of food.

Snigdha
Unctuous nature.

Sthir
Firm, of less mobility.

Sangrahe
Substance which binds stool or constipation causing.

Sransan
Helps to excrete hard stoolie, constipation reliever.

Stambham
Stops oozing & visarjan and being astringent cures constipation.

Supral
Increases quality of semen.

Suksma
Which can enter the body through pores.

Srit seat
After boiling the cool water is called srit seat.

Satak
100 years old ghee. It is also known as Kumbhgrrit .

Tarpak Kapha
Satisfying natured kapha.

Tiksanta
Sharpness

Tamsik form
Lazy or lethargic, deluded or prove to attachment.

Takra
Buttermilk made by churning curd with one fourth water.

Udana
Rising air.

Usna
Hot, fiery natured.

Uttarayana
Sun's northern hemispherical inclined transit-period.

Udswit
Quantity of water in curd is half at the churning time.

Vata
It is one of the Tridosas. It is a combination of elements Air & Space. It is concerned with the movement, breathing, natural urges, secretions, fears & anxiety.

Vayu
It is known as one of the five elements. It is concerned with the sense of touch related to skin by the action of holding it.

VriksAyurved
Way of treating the disorder in botanical growth according Ayurved.

Vaajikaran Tantra
Treating the genital or sex related problems.

Vaisesik
Another branch of vedic philosophical school.

Vayavya diet
Diet having vayu as dominant element.

Vayana
Diffused air through out the body.

Visadata
Non-oily nature.

Visragandhita
Fleshy smell.

Virecan
Induced vomiting as treatment.

Vidahi
causing burning sensation.

Vikashi
Ealming limbs and ligaments of the joints

Visarg
Due to the plenty of herbs and plants as well as cooling process the daksinayan is also known as visarg.

Vandranstra
Period between two seasons, Prone to various diseases i.e. last 8 days of kartik and first 8 days of aghan.
